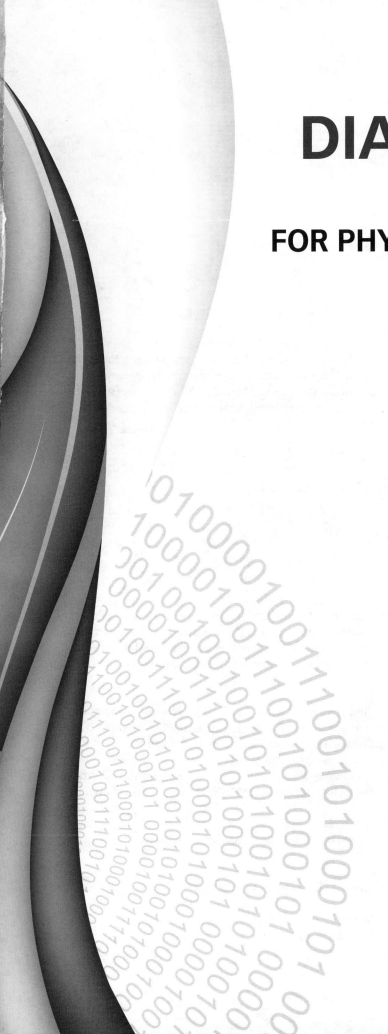

DIAGNOSTIC CODING
FOR PHYSICIAN SERVICES:
ICD-10-CM

2014 Edition

Anita C. Hazelwood,
MLS, RHIA, FAHIMA

Carol A. Venable,
MPH, RHIA, FAHIMA

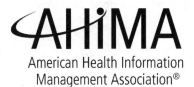

D1466406

American Health Information
Management Association®

ISBN: 978-1-58426-076-9
AHIMA Product No.: AC201213

Angie Comfort, RHIT, CDIP, CCS, Director, HIM Practice Excellence
Jessica Block, MA, Assistant Editor
Kathryn DeVault, RHIA, CCS, CCS-P, Director, HIM Practice Excellence
Megan Grennan, Production Development Editor
Jason O. Malley, Director, Creative Content Development
Pamela Woolf, Managing Editor

The websites listed in this book were current and valid as of the date of publication. However, webpage addresses and the information on them may change at any time. The user is encouraged to perform his or her own general web searches to locate any site addresses listed here that are no longer valid.

CPT® is a registered trademark of the American Medical Association. All other copyrights and trademarks mentioned in this book are the possession of their respective owners. AHIMA makes no claim of ownership by mentioning products that contain such marks.

For more information about AHIMA Press publications, including updates, visit http://www.ahima.org/publications/updates.aspx

American Health Information Management Association
233 North Michigan Avenue, 21st Floor
Chicago, Illinois 60601-5809
ahima.org

Contents

About the Authors

Carol A. Venable, MPH, RHIA, FAHIMA, is the former HIM department head and professor at the University of Louisiana at Lafayette. Anita C. Hazelwood, MLS, RHIA, FAHIMA, is the current director of the program and a professor at the same university. Their book, *ICD-10-CM and ICD-10-PCS Preview*, was first published by AHIMA in 2003 and was updated in 2004, 2008, and 2013. They are also coauthors of *Certified Coding Specialist-Physician Based (CCSP)*.

Both authors are AHIMA approved ICD-10-CM and ICD-10-PCS trainers and have conducted numerous coding workshops at the local, state, and national levels. They have published articles in *Educational Perspectives in Health Information Management* and in the *Journal of AHIMA*.

Active volunteers of AHIMA, Ms. Venable and Ms. Hazelwood have served in various capacities and on committees.

Preface

The coding process requires a range of skills that combine knowledge and practice. *Diagnostic Coding for Physician Services: ICD-10-CM* is designed to provide a comprehensive text for students and physician-based coding personnel. It introduces the basic principles and conventions of ICD-10-CM coding, illustrates the application of coding principles with examples and exercises based on actual case documentation, and teaches students and physician-based coding personnel how to analyze clinical data for the purposes of coding and reimbursement.

Acknowledgments

The authors are grateful for the contributions of Lou Ann Schraffenberger, and they wish to thank Debra Moore, CCS, CPC, for her review of the text.

Organization of the Book

Each of the chapters in the book covers coding rules and guidelines as well as numerous coding exercises found in ICD-10-CM.

Chapter 1, Introduction to ICD-10-CM, provides a general overview of coding and classification systems and presents the basic characteristics, conventions, and principles of coding. The chapter illustrates how to read and interpret documentation in the medical record and understand the basic steps and rules to follow for coding diagnoses. It also presents current, approved coding guidelines for assigning and sequencing accurate diagnosis codes.

Chapter 2, Infectious and Parasitic Diseases, presents general information on basic laboratory tests that physicians might order and reviews common microorganisms. Guidelines for coding infectious and parasitic conditions are covered.

Chapter 3, Neoplasms, describes the current, approved ICD-10-CM coding guidelines to follow when assigning and sequencing codes for diagnoses related to neoplasms. It also explains how to use the Neoplasm Table and the terms that apply to each of its columns.

Chapter 4, Diseases of the Blood and Blood-Forming Organs, presents coding rules related to diseases of the blood and blood-forming organs. Guidelines for assigning codes for anemia, coagulation defects, hemorrhagic conditions, and diseases of the white blood cells are included.

Chapter 5, Endocrine, Nutritional, and Metabolic Diseases, covers the most commonly diagnosed endocrine, nutritional, metabolic, and immunity disorders, such as diabetes mellitus, hypoglycemia, and thyroid disorders.

Chapter 6, Mental, Behavioral, and Neurodevelopmental Disorders, discusses the most common mental disorders and the correct way to assign codes for these types of diagnoses. Coding guidelines for substance abuse are also reviewed.

Chapter 7, Diseases of the Nervous System, discusses common disorders of the nervous system and describes the current, approved guidelines coders should follow when assigning and sequencing codes for diagnoses related to the nervous system.

Chapter 8, Diseases of the Eye and Adnexa, includes common diseases of the eye and adnexa, such as conjunctivitis, glaucoma, and cataracts.

Chapter 9, Diseases of Ear and Mastoid Process, includes common diseases of the ear and mastoid process, such as otitis media.

Chapter 10, Diseases of the Circulatory System, discusses the most common disorders of the circulatory system and the current, approved guidelines coders should follow when assigning and sequencing codes for these diagnoses.

Chapter 11, Diseases of the Respiratory System, discusses common disorders of the respiratory system and explains the current, approved guidelines coders should follow when assigning and sequencing codes for diagnoses related to this organ system.

Chapter 12, Diseases of the Digestive System, discusses the major disorders of the digestive system and the approved guidelines coders should follow when assigning and sequencing codes related to this organ system.

Chapter 13, Diseases of the Skin and Subcutaneous Tissue, classifies diagnoses for disorders of the skin and subcutaneous tissue and provides guidelines for the proper coding and sequencing of diagnoses related to these conditions.

Chapter 14, Diseases of the Musculoskeletal System and Connective Tissue, provides information on the most common disorders related to the musculoskeletal system.

Chapter 15, Diseases of the Genitourinary System, covers the most common disorders of the genitourinary system and provides coding guidelines for assigning and sequencing codes for diagnoses related to this organ system.

Chapter 16, Complications of Pregnancy, Childbirth, and the Puerperium, clarifies the coding rules that apply to pregnancy, delivery, and the postpartum period.

Chapter 17, Certain Conditions Originating in the Perinatal Period: Congenital Malformations, Deformations, and Chromosomal Abnormalities, discusses the major anomalies and perinatal conditions that affect newborns. Definitions of congenital anomalies and perinatal conditions are reviewed.

Chapter 18, Symptoms, Signs, and Abnormal Clinical and Laboratory Findings, discusses the current, approved guidelines coders should follow when assigning and sequencing codes for diagnoses related to signs, symptoms, and ill-defined conditions.

Chapter 19, Injury, Poisonings, and Adverse Effects, covers a wide variety of injuries and also includes information on poisoning and adverse reactions to drugs. Coding guidelines for the reporting and sequencing of diagnoses are thoroughly reviewed.

Chapter 20, Complications of Surgical and Medical Care, provides an overview of complications of care that are not classified in other chapters in the ICD-10-CM codebook. A discussion of what constitutes postoperative complications is included.

Chapter 21, Factors Influencing Health Status and Contact with Health Services, includes coding guidelines for situations when it is appropriate to use a Z code. Some of the most commonly used Z codes are reviewed.

Chapter 22, Challenges of Compliance and Ethical Coding, identifies the legislation related to fraud and abuse as well as components of compliance plans for healthcare organizations.

Chapter 23, Training and Implementation of ICD-10-CM, identifies the challenges faced in the training and implementation phases of ICD-10-CM and the impact on the health information, IT, and other departments in organizations.

The index and appendices at the back of the book make information readily accessible and provide additional resources for students and physician-based coders.

This book must be used with the 2014 edition of *ICD-10-CM* (code changes effective October 1, 2014).

Additional Practice

AHIMA's publication, *Clinical Coding Workout: Practice Exercises for Skill Development* (AHIMA product numbers AC201514, with answers, and AC201614, without answers), is an excellent follow-up resource after the coder completes *Diagnostic Coding for Physician Services: ICD-10-CM*. *Clinical Coding Workout: Practice Exercises for Skill Development* is a perfect teaching tool for coders wanting to sharpen their ability to make critical coding decisions. The book contains beginning through advanced practice exercises, including case studies that help students and coders alike understand what they need to know when it comes to correct coding practices and procedures. The case studies require users to make the kinds of decisions that coding professionals must make every day on the job.

Introduction to ICD-10-CM

Chapter 1

OBJECTIVES

After completing this lesson, you should be able to do the following:

- Explain the purpose of classification and coding systems
- Identify the basic characteristics, conventions, symbols, and principles of the ICD-10-CM classification systems
- Understand the basic steps and rules to follow for the coding of diagnoses
- Apply knowledge of current ICD-10-CM coding guidelines for the assignment and sequencing of codes for diagnoses

Introduction to ICD-10-CM

Healthcare data in the form of ICD-10-CM diagnostic codes are collected and reported for patients receiving medical care in all settings: inpatient, ambulatory care surgery, observation, outpatient, rehabilitation, skilled nursing, physician office, and home health, for example. The clinical health information is converted into coded data that are used for multiple purposes, including:

- Trending
- Planning
- Making comparisons
- Determining reimbursement
- Determining appropriate levels of service
- Justifying levels of service
- Measuring quality of care
- Measuring severity of illness
- Measuring intensity of service

The process of collecting and reporting these data is complex, and careful documentation is critical for accurate and complete data collection. The source document—the health record—must describe the encounter both qualitatively and quantitatively and must specify the reason for the visit (such as the condition, symptom, or diagnosis requiring attention) and the services provided.

Definition of Coding

In its simplest form, coding is the transformation of verbal descriptions into numbers. We are all familiar with this task, because we use codes every day to carry out simple business and personal transactions. For example, a zip code transforms a geographical location into numbers. In the healthcare arena, specific codes describe diseases, injuries, and procedures. Whereas assigning zip code is a rather simple task, assigning diagnostic and procedural codes is a detailed process that requires a thorough knowledge of medical terminology, anatomy, and pathophysiology.

The method of classifying diseases and procedures has evolved through the years into a sophisticated system that can track general and nonspecific conditions, such as abdominal pain, to specific diagnoses, such as acute cholecystitis with cholelithiasis. Hospitals have used coding systems to categorize diagnoses and procedures for many years. Since the 1980s, Medicare has required physicians to submit the appropriate diagnostic codes to identify the reason for a patient visit or encounter, such as a diagnosis (hypertension) or a symptom (chest pain).

Development of the Coding System

Healthcare providers, such as physicians and hospitals, index healthcare data by referring and adhering to a classification system published by the US Department of Health and Human Services (HHS): the *International Classification of Diseases, Ninth Revision, Clinical Modification (ICD-10-CM)*. As the title indicates, this coding system has been revised 10 times, signifying that it has been in use for many years.

The notion of using classification systems can be traced back to the time of the ancient Greeks. In the 17th century, English statistician John Graunt developed the *London Bills of Mortality*, which was the first attempt to identify the proportion of children who died before reaching age six. In 1838, William Farr, registrar general of England, developed a system to classify deaths. And in 1893, a French physician, Jacques Bertillon, unveiled the *Bertillon Classification of Causes of Death* at the International Statistical Institute in Chicago.

Several countries adopted Bertillon's system; in 1898, the American Public Health Association (APHA) recommended that the registrars of Canada, Mexico, and the United States also adopt it. In addition, APHA recommended revising the system every 10 years to remain current with medical practice. The first international conference to revise the *International Classification of Causes of Death* was convened in 1900, and the system has been revised every 10 years thereafter. At the time of the first conference, the classification system was contained in one book, which included an Alphabetic Index and a Tabular List. As can be imagined, the book was quite small in comparison with current coding manuals.

Early revisions of the classification system involved only minor changes; however, the sixth revision brought drastic changes, and the publication was expanded to two volumes. That revision included morbidity and mortality conditions, and its title was modified to reflect these changes: *Manual of International Statistical Classification of Diseases, Injuries and Causes of Death (ICD)*. Prior to the sixth revision, responsibility for ICD revisions fell to the Mixed Commission, a group composed of representatives from the International Statistical Institute and the Health Organization of the League of Nations. In 1948, the World Health Organization (WHO), headquartered in Geneva, Switzerland, assumed responsibility for preparing and publishing the revisions to the ICD code book. WHO sponsored the seventh and eighth revisions in 1957 and 1968, respectively.

The entire history of the ICD coding system emphasizes the determination of many people to provide an international classification system for compiling and presenting statistical data. ICD is currently the most widely used statistical classification system in the world.

After WHO published the ninth revision of the ICD system in 1978, the United States modified it to meet the needs of American hospitals and called it *International Classification of Diseases, Ninth*

Revision, Clinical Modification (ICD-9-CM). The ninth revision expanded the book to three volumes and introduced a fifth-digit subclassification.

A tenth revision of the ICD system has been developed at the international level and adapted for use in the United States. The actual implementation date for ICD-10-CM is October 1, 2014.

To ensure accurate coding, all ICD-10-CM code books must be updated yearly with code revisions. In addition, all coding software (encoders, electronic coding software, electronic coding references, and such) must be updated.

General Coding Guidelines

To facilitate and standardize physician office coding, official coding guidelines were developed by CMS, AHA, AHIMA, and NCHS. Throughout this book, coding guidelines are presented for specific diseases and body systems. The most recent official coding guidelines for outpatient services, including physician offices, are provided in the *ICD-10-CM Official Guidelines for Coding and Reporting 2013.* The most current version of these guidelines is available online. A summary of these guidelines follows:

- Use the appropriate code or codes from A00.00–T88.9 and Z00–Z99.8 to identify diagnoses, symptoms, conditions, problems, complaints, or other reason(s) for the encounter or visit.

- ICD-10-CM is composed of codes with three, four, five, six, or seven characters. A three-digit character is used as the heading of a category of codes that may be further subdivided with fourth, fifth, sixth, and seventh characters to provide greater specificity.

  Use a three-character code only when it is not further subdivided. A code is considered invalid when it has not been coded to the full number of characters required for that code.

  > **EXAMPLE:** E11 Incorrect code assignment
  >
  > E11.0 Incorrect code assignment
  >
  > E11.01 Correct code assignment

  It is recognized that a specific diagnosis may not be known at the time of an initial office visit; however, this is not an acceptable reason for submitting a three digit code when a fourth, fifth, sixth, or seventh character code is more appropriate.

- First list the ICD-10-CM code for the diagnosis, condition, problem, or other reason for the encounter or visit shown in the health record to be chiefly responsible for the services provided; then list additional codes that describe any coexisting conditions.

  > **EXAMPLE:** Patient was seen in the physician's office with a complaint of polyuria and polydipsia. During the visit, the patient's hypertension was evaluated and the prescription refilled. The first code listed may be either the polyuria or the polydipsia, because this was the primary reason for the visit, followed by a code for the hypertension.

- At the time of discharge, code any condition described as *impending* or *threatened* according to the following guidelines:

  - Code a confirmed diagnosis if the condition did occur.
  - If the condition did not occur, refer to the Alphabetic Index and check for a subentry term for impending or threatened.
  - Main entry terms impending and threatened may also be referenced for a code assignment. Assign the code indicated if there is a subterm listed. If there are no subterms listed, the code for the existing underlying condition(s) should be coded and not the condition identified as impending or threatened.

- Codes that describe symptoms and signs, as opposed to diagnoses, are acceptable for reporting purposes when a diagnosis has not been established or confirmed by the physician. Chapter 18, Symptoms, Signs, and Abnormal Clinical and Laboratory Findings not elsewhere classified, lists many but not all codes for symptoms. Some signs and symptoms are routinely associated with a given disease process and should not be assigned as additional codes unless one is specifically instructed to do so. Any signs/symptoms that are not routinely associated with a disease should be coded, if present.
- ICD-10-CM provides codes to deal with encounters for circumstances other than a disease or injury. Chapter 21 of ICD-10-CM, Factors influencing health status and contact with health services (Z00–Z99), deals with occasions when circumstances other than a disease or injury are recorded as diagnoses or problems.
- The etiology or manifestation convention requires the use of two codes to completely describe a single condition that may affect multiple body systems. There are single conditions that may also require the use of more than one code. Multiple codes may be needed for sequelae, complication codes, and obstetric codes in order to fully describe a condition.

    In the Tabular List, if the following instructions are included, it may be necessary to use an additional code(s):

    ▸ "Use additional code" note may be found listed under certain codes that are not part of an etiology or manifestation pair, but the use of a secondary code may be necessary to fully describe a condition or disease process. If this is the case, a secondary code should be added.

    ▸ "Code first" notes may also be listed under certain codes that are not specifically manifestation codes but may indicate an underlying cause. When this "Code first" note is present along with an underlying condition, the underlying condition should be coded and sequenced first.

    ▸ "Code, if applicable, any causal condition first" note indicates that this code may be assigned as a principal diagnosis when the causal condition is not known or applicable. In the event that the causal condition is known, then the code for that condition should be listed as the first listed diagnosis.

- Code all documented conditions that coexist at the time of the encounter or visit and that require or affect patient treatment or management. Do not code conditions that were treated previously and no longer exist. However, history codes (Z80–Z87) may be used as secondary codes when the historical condition or family history has an impact on current care or influences treatment.
- For patients receiving diagnostic services only during an encounter or visit, sequence first the diagnosis, condition, problem, or other reason for the encounter or visit shown in the health record to be chiefly responsible for the outpatient services provided during the encounter or visit. Codes for other diagnoses (for example, chronic conditions) may be sequenced as additional diagnoses.
- For patients receiving therapeutic services only during an encounter or visit, sequence first the diagnosis, condition, problem, or other reason for the encounter or visit shown in the health record to be chiefly responsible for the outpatient services provided during the encounter or visit. Codes for other diagnoses (for example, chronic conditions) may be sequenced as additional diagnoses. There is one exception: for patients receiving chemotherapy or radiation therapy, list first the appropriate Z code that identifies the service and then the diagnosis or problem for which the service is being performed.
- For patients receiving preoperative evaluations only, sequence a code from category Z01.818, Encounter for other preprocedural examination, to describe the preoperative consultations.

Assign a code for the condition to describe the reason for the surgery as an additional diagnosis. Also code any findings related to the preoperative evaluation.

- For ambulatory surgery, code the diagnosis for which the surgery was performed. When the postoperative diagnosis is known to be different from the preoperative diagnosis at the time the diagnosis is confirmed, select the postoperative diagnosis for coding, because it is the most definitive one.

- For routine outpatient prenatal visits when no complications are present, code Z34.00, Encounter for supervision of other normal pregnancy, unspecified trimester, should be used as the first list diagnosis. These codes should not be used in conjunction with the codes in Chapter 15.

- Acute and chronic conditions: In the event that a condition is described as both acute (or subacute) and chronic and the Alphabetic Index lists separate subentries at the same indentation level, then both conditions should be coded, with the acute code listed first.

- A combination code is a single code used to identify two diagnoses, or a diagnosis with a manifestation, or a diagnosis with a listed complication. Combination codes are identified by referring to subterms in the Alphabetic Index along with reading any Includes or Excludes notes in the Tabular List. A combination code should only be assigned when the code fully identifies the diagnostic condition or when the Alphabetic Index directs the coder to use this code.

- A sequela is defined as the residual condition produced after the acute phase of an injury or illness has past (late effect). There is no time limit for when a sequela code can be used. In some cases, the residual condition may be apparent early, or it may occur months or even years later. In order to properly code a sequela, two codes are generally required—the nature or condition of the sequela is sequenced first, with the sequela code being sequenced second.

  There is an exception to the above rule when the sequela is followed by a manifestation code identified in the Tabular List and code title, or when the sequela code has been expanded to include the manifestation(s). A code for the acute phase of an injury or illness that ultimately led to the sequela is never to be used with a code for the sequela.

  Documentation in the health record may include the following terms and phrases to indicate a sequela:

  ▸ Residuals of
  ▸ Old
  ▸ Sequela of
  ▸ Late
  ▸ Due to a previous illness or injury
  ▸ Following a previous illness or injury

- In ICD-10-CM, some codes indicate laterality, which specifies whether the condition or injury occurred on the right or left side or bilaterally. If the condition is bilateral, but there are no codes specified for this, use separate codes for both the right and left sides. If the specific site is not specified anywhere in the patient's record, assign the code for an unspecified side.

- When coding syndromes in ICD-10-CM, follow the Alphabetic Index guidance. If the Alphabetic Index does not offer any specific guidance, assign codes for any manifestations of the syndrome that have been documented. Additional codes for manifestations that were not an integral part of a disease process can also be assigned when the condition does not have a unique code.

- When coding complications of care, there must be a cause-and-effect relationship that exists between the care that is provided and the condition. There should also be an indication in the documentation that this is in fact a complication. The provider may be queried for further clarification if the complication is not clearly documented.

- If a physician provides a borderline diagnosis, then code the diagnosis as confirmed, unless the classification provides a specific entry and code (for example, borderline diabetes). If the documentation is not clear regarding a borderline diagnosis, the provider should be queried for further clarification.

Characteristics and Conventions of ICD-10-CM

ICD-10-CM conventions are incorporated within both the Tabular List and Alphabetical Index as instructional notes.

Tabular List of Diseases and Injuries

The Tabular List is a chronological list of codes divided into chapters that are based on condition or body system. Codes in this list appear in numerical order. Code numbers and corresponding titles appear in the Tabular List in bold print. It also includes instructional notes applying to sections, categories, or subcategories.

Classification of Diseases and Injuries

The main classification of Diseases and Injuries contains 21 chapters that classify conditions according to etiology (cause of disease) or by a specific anatomical (body) system.

The 21 chapters of the ICD-10-CM classification system are listed here:

1. Certain infectious and parasitic diseases (A00–B99)
2. Neoplasms (C00–D49)
3. Diseases of the blood and blood-forming organs and certain disorders involving the immune mechanism (D50–D89)
4. Endocrine, nutritional, and metabolic disorders (E00–E89)
5. Mental, behavioral, and neurodevelopmental disorders (F01–F99)
6. Diseases of the nervous system (G00–G99)
7. Diseases of the eye and adnexa (H00–H59)
8. Diseases of the ear and mastoid process (H60–H95)
9. Diseases of the circulatory system (I00–I99)
10. Diseases of the respiratory system (J00–J99)
11. Diseases of the digestive system (K00–K95)
12. Diseases of the skin and subcutaneous tissue (L00–L99)
13. Diseases of the musculoskeletal system and connective tissue (M00–M99)
14. Diseases of the genitourinary system (N00–N99)
15. Pregnancy, childbirth, and the puerperium (O00–O9A)
16. Certain conditions originating in the perinatal period (P00–P96)
17. Congenital malformations, deformations, and chromosomal abnormalities (Q00–Q99)
18. Symptoms, signs, and abnormal clinical and laboratory findings, not elsewhere classified (R00–R99)
19. Injury, poisoning, and certain other consequences of external causes (S00–T88)

20. External causes of morbidity (V00–Y99)
21. Factors influencing health status and contact with health services (Z00–Z99)

Format and Code Structure

The format and structure of ICD-10-CM contains sections, categories, subcategories, subclassifications, and codes. All category codes contain three characters (letters or numbers) and maybe further subdivided with fourth, fifth, or sixth characters. In some cases, a seventh character or extension may also be used. A code without the applicable number of characters is considered to be an invalid code.

ICD-10-CM uses a placeholder character X. The X is used as a fifth character placeholder in certain six character codes allows for future expansion. Certain ICD-10-CM categories have applicable seventh characters, which must be in the seventh character space. If a code does not have six characters, placeholders are used to fill the empty spaces.

Each chapter is structured into the following subdivisions:

- Sections
- Categories
- Subcategories
- Subclassifications

Sections

A section consists of a group of three character categories that represents a single disease entity or a group of similar or closely related conditions; for example, Disorders of the Thyroid Gland (E00–E07).

Categories

An individual three character category represents a single disease entity or a group of similar or closely related conditions; for example, E20, Hypoparathyroidism.

Subcategories

The fourth character subcategory code numbers provide more specificity or information regarding the etiology (cause), site, or manifestation (characteristic signs, symptoms, or secondary processes) of an illness.

Subclassifications

In some cases, fourth character subcategories have been expanded to the fifth, sixth, or seventh character level to provide even greater specificity. In addition, some categories have a seventh character extension that is required for all codes in the category. These seventh character extensions must always be the last character in the code number. Characters for categories, subcategories, and codes may be either a number or a letter.

EXAMPLE: C44 Other and unspecified malignant neoplasms of skin

C44.1 Other and unspecified malignant neoplasm of skin of eyelid, including canthus

C44.10 Unspecified malignant neoplasm of skin of eyelid, including canthus

C44.101 Unspecified malignant neoplasm of skin of unspecified eyelid, including canthus

Alphabetic Index to Diseases

The Alphabetic Index is an alphabetical list of terms and their corresponding codes. The Alphabetic Index consists of the following: the Index to Diseases and Injuries, the Neoplasm Table, the Table of Drugs and Chemicals, and the Index to External Causes.

Main Terms

Printed in boldface type, the main terms are set flush with the left margin of each column for easy reference and begin with a capital letter. Main terms may represent

- Diseases (for example, influenza, bronchitis)
- Conditions (for example, fatigue, fracture, injury)
- Nouns (for example, disease, disturbance, syndrome)
- Adjectives (for example, double, large, kinking)

Subterms

Some main terms are followed by a list of indented subterms (modifiers) that affect the selection of an appropriate code for a given diagnosis. The subterms form individual line entries arranged in alphabetical order and printed in regular type, beginning with a lowercase letter. Subterms are indented one standard indentation to the right under the main term. They describe essential differences in site, cause, or clinical type. More specific subterms are indented farther to the right, as needed, indented one standard indentation after the preceding subterm, and listed in alphabetical order. A dash (-) at the end of an index entry indicates that there are additional characters required.

Carryover Lines

Carryover lines are needed because there is a limit to the number of words that can fit on a single line of print in the Index to Diseases and Injuries. Carryover lines are indented two standard indent spaces from the preceding line.

Nonessential Modifiers

A series of terms in parentheses, called nonessential modifiers, sometimes directly follows a main term or subterm. The presence or absence of nonessential modifiers in the diagnosis has no effect on the selection of the code listed for that main term or subterm.

> **EXAMPLE:** Pneumonia (acute) (double) (migratory) (purulent) (septic) (unresolved) J18.9

Appendices

The Alphabetic Index contains the following appendices:

Neoplasm Table: The Neoplasm Table provides the proper code based on histology of the neoplasm and site.

Table of Drugs and Chemicals: The Table of Drugs and Chemicals is an alphabetical listing of drugs and the specific codes that identify the drug and the intent. No additional external cause or injury and poisoning code is assigned in ICD-10-CM.

Index to External Causes: The Index to External Causes of Injury is arranged in alphabetic order by main term indicating the event.

Conventions in ICD-10-CM

To assign diagnostic codes accurately, a thorough understanding of ICD-10-CM conventions is necessary, including those for cross-references and instructional notations.

Cross-References

Cross references in the Alphabetic Index are directions to look elsewhere in the code book before a code is assigned. The following subsections discuss two types of cross-reference terms: *see*, and *see also*.

See: The *see* cross-reference points to an alternative term. This mandatory instruction must be followed to ensure accurate assignment of ICD-10-CM codes.

> **EXAMPLE:**   Hemangioblastoma—*See* Neoplasm, connective tissue, uncertain behavior

See Also: The second type of cross-reference direction is *see also*. This instruction requires a review of another main term in the Index when all the needed information cannot be found under the first main term.

> **EXAMPLE:**   Impaction, impacted
>
> bowel, colon, rectum (*See also* Impaction, fecal)

Conventions and Notes

ICD-10-CM contains the following conventions and notes: includes notes, inclusion terms, excludes notes, and instructional notes.

Includes Notes

Includes notes are used throughout the Tabular List and appear immediately under a three character code title to further define or provide an example of the content of the category.

> **EXAMPLE:**   Chapter 1, Certain Infectious and Parasitic Diseases (A00–B99)
>
> Includes: diseases generally recognized as communicable or transmissible

Inclusion Terms: A list of terms is included under some codes, and these terms are the conditions for which that code is to be used. These terms may be synonymous to the code title. With other specified codes, the terms are a listing of the various conditions assigned to that code. The list of inclusion terms is not necessarily exhaustive, as additional terms found only in the Alphabetic Index may also be coded.

Excludes Notes

In ICD-10-CM, there are two types of excludes notes. Each type of excludes note has a different definition for its use, but they are all similar, in that they indicate that codes excluded from each other are also independent of each other.

Excludes 1: An Excludes 1 note is a pure excludes note and means that the condition is "not listed here," and should never be used at the same time as the code above the Excludes 1 note. This note is used when two conditions cannot occur together, such as a congenital form versus an acquired form of the same condition.

> **EXAMPLE:**   Q21 Congenital malformation of cardiac septa
>
> Excludes 1 – acquired cardiac septal defect (I51.0)

Excludes 2: An Excludes 2 note means "not included here." An Excludes 2 note indicates that the condition excluded is not part of the condition represented by the code; however, a patient may have both conditions at the same time. When an Excludes 2 note appears under a code, it is acceptable to use both the code and the excludes note together, when appropriate.

> **EXAMPLE:**   F94.2 Disinhibited attachment disorder of childhood
>
> Excludes 2 – Asperger's syndrome (F84.5)

In this example, the Excludes 2 note indicates that if a patient has both a disinhibited attachment disorder of childhood and Asperger's syndrome, both conditions may be coded.

Multiple Code Assignment

The use of more than one code to fully identify a given condition is often necessary in ICD-10-CM coding. In such cases, one code describes the cause, or etiology, of the condition; and the other, the manifestation(s). Several instructional notations alert coders that the assignment of more than one code is required. Instructions for sequencing and coordinating multiple codes also should be followed.

Code First/Use Additional Code

Code first/use additional code notes are in red type and provide sequencing instruction for the coder. They can appear independently of each other or to designate certain etiology or manifestation paired codes. These types of instructions signal the coder that an additional code needs to be reported in order to provide a more complete picture of that diagnosis.

In etiology or manifestation coding, ICD-10-CM requires that the underlying condition be sequenced first, followed by the manifestation. In this type of situation, codes with "In disease classified elsewhere" in the code description are never used as the first-listed diagnosis code but rather must be sequenced after the code for the underlying condition.

> **EXAMPLE:** F01 Vascular dementia
>
> Code first underlying physiological condition or sequelae of cerebrovascular disease

> **EXAMPLE:** F01.51 Vascular dementia with behavioral disturbance
>
> Use additional code, if applicable, to identify wandering in vascular dementia (Z91.83)

Code Also

A code also note warns the coder that more than one code may be required to fully describe the condition. In these cases, code sequencing is discretionary. These coding notes also appear in red type.

> **EXAMPLE:** G47.01 Insomnia due to medical condition
>
> Code also associated medical condition

Connecting Words

The following are examples of subterms listed in the Alphabetic Index that indicate a relationship between the main term or a subterm and an associated condition or etiology:

- Associated with
- Due to
- In
- With

The connecting words "with" and "without" are sequenced before all other subterms below the main term. The word "with" should be interpreted to mean "associated with" or "due to" when it appears in a code title, the Alphabetic Index, or an instructional note in the Tabular List. Other connecting words are listed in alphabetical order.

Abbreviations, Punctuation, and Symbols

ICD-10-CM uses a variety of symbols, punctuation, and abbreviations, which are discussed in the following paragraphs.

Abbreviations

Two abbreviations related to coding that are used in ICD-10-CM are NEC, for codes that are not elsewhere classifiable, and NOS, for codes not otherwise specified.

NEC: Not Elsewhere Classifiable

NEC serves two purposes. First, it can be used with ill-defined terms listed in the Tabular List to warn the coder that specified forms of the condition are classified differently. The codes given for such terms should be used only when more precise information is unavailable.

Second, NEC can be used with terms for which a more specific code is unavailable, even though the diagnostic statement is specific.

NOS: Not Otherwise Specified

The equivalent of unspecified, NOS (not otherwise specified) is used in both the Tabular List and the Alphabetic Index. Codes describing NOS conditions are assigned only when the diagnostic statement or the health record does not provide enough information to use more specific codes.

Punctuation

ICD-10-CM uses three punctuation marks with specialized meanings. It should be noted that some publishers of ICD-10-CM have elected not to use certain punctuation marks.

Parentheses ( )

Parentheses enclose supplementary words or explanatory information that may or may not be present in the statement of a diagnosis or procedure. They do not affect the code number assigned to the case. Terms in parentheses are considered nonessential modifiers, and are used in both the Tabular List and Alphabetic Index.

Square Brackets [ ]

Square brackets are used to enclose synonyms, alternative wordings, abbreviations, and explanatory phrases. In effect, they are similar to parentheses in that they are not required as part of the diagnostic statement. Square brackets are used only in the Tabular List.

Colon :

The colon is used in the Tabular List after an incomplete term that needs one or more of the modifiers that follow, so that it can be assigned to a given category or code.

Relational Terms

The word "and" should be interpreted to mean either "and" or "or" when it appears in a title.

Use of the Health Record in the Coding Process

The coding process for each physician's office should be organized to address the following:

- Review of the health record
- Selection of codes significant for the current episode of care

- Criteria for the sequencing of diagnostic and procedural codes
- Interaction with physician(s) regarding documentation issues
- Generic coding guidelines
- System-specific coding guidelines for different body systems
- Reimbursement requirements

These elements of the process should be documented in a coding policy and procedure manual developed jointly by the health information office manager and the physician(s). In addition, the advice and support of any and all users of encoded medical data should be sought. The criteria should address the comprehensive, and sometimes unique, data needs of the office practice; local, state, and national reporting requirements; third-party reimbursement requirements; and professional standards of care as determined by the physician(s).

Coding policies and procedures should be continuously assessed and updated using *ICD-10-CM's Official Guidelines for Coding and Reporting* and AHA's ICD-10-CM/PCS *Coding Clinic.*

After a thorough review of the record has been completed, the coder must uniformly apply coding principles and official coding guidelines to report the appropriate diagnoses. In almost all instances, the coder can confidently identify the principal diagnosis after carefully reviewing the documentation. However, problems may be encountered in poorly or inconsistently documented records. In such instances, documentation deficiencies should be discussed with the physician(s).

Basic Steps in ICD-10-CM Coding

The following basic steps must be followed in ICD-10-CM coding after determining the diagnoses that must be coded. To code each disease or condition completely and accurately, the coder should

- Identify all main terms included in the diagnostic statement(s).
- Locate each main term in the Alphabetic Index.
- Refer to any subterms indented under the main term. The subterms form individual line entries and describe essential differences by site, etiology, or clinical type.
- Follow cross-reference instructions when the needed code is not located under the first main term consulted.
- Verify the code selected in the Tabular List or notes in the Tabular List.
- Assign codes to their highest level of specificity up to a total of seven characters if applicable.
- Continue coding the diagnostic statement until all the component elements are fully identified.

Chapter 1: ICD-10-CM Exercises

Select the correct multiple choice answer:

1. Physicians use ICD-10-CM to describe _____?
   a. Diagnoses
   b. Procedures
   c. Services
   d. Supplies

2. Which of the following codes represents a subclassification?
   a. A06.4
   b. E11
   c. D49.89
   d. B20

3. Which of the following codes represents a subclassification?
   a. C83.8
   b. I10
   c. B60.10
   d. E15

4. Seventh characters in the Injury, Poisoning, and Certain Other Consequences of External Causes refer to:
   a. Initial encounters, subsequent encounters, or a sequel
   b. Identifying the specific fetus in cases of multiple gestations
   c. Mild, moderate, severe, or intermediate stage of disease
   d. With or without tophus

Review the following diagnoses and underline the main term:

5. Tension headache

6. Irregular menstruation

7. Diverticula of cecum

8. Congestive heart failure

9. Ewing's sarcoma

10. Allergic gastroenteritis

11. Female infertility

12. Erb's palsy

13. Olfactory hallucination

14. Pyogenic arthritis

Answer the following questions:

15. According to the Excludes 1 note under category D89, what conditions are excluded?

Continued

16. According to the Excludes 2 note under category D89, what condition is listed?

_____

17. What type of instructional note is listed below code J10.0?

_____

18. According to the note under P08.1, how is an exceptionally large baby defined?

_____

19. According to the inclusion note under category G50, what condition is included?

_____

20. What notation is located under category I50?

_____

Review the following statements and assign the appropriate codes:

21. Localized osteoarthritis of right knee

22. Bleeding esophageal varices in liver cirrhosis

23. Urinary tract infection due to Shiga toxin-producing *Escherichia coli* (*E. coli*) O157

24. Bronchiolitis due to respiratory syncytial virus

25. Diabetic neuropathy

26. Newborn purpura

27. Pneumonia due to *Klebsiella* (pneumoniae)

28. Viral encephalitis due to a tick bite

29. Trench fever

30. Microscopic hematuria

Infectious and Parasitic Diseases

OBJECTIVES

After completing this lesson, you should be able to do the following:

- Apply knowledge of current ICD-10-CM coding guidelines to assign and sequence accurate codes for infectious and parasitic diseases
- Generally understand the basic laboratory tests performed to assist physicians in the diagnosis and treatment of infectious diseases
- Identify the general categories of microorganisms that cause infections
- Be able to properly code bacteremia, septicemia, SIRS, and septic shock

ICD-10-CM

Chapter 1 of the ICD-10-CM code book includes diseases recognized as communicable or transmissible and some diseases of unknown, but possibly infectious, origin. The infectious and parasitic diseases incorporated within Chapter 1 are classified primarily by organism. Noncommunicable diseases are classified by site to other chapters in the code book. Physicians of all specialties use these codes to identify infections that affect any body system. The infectious and parasitic diseases chapter is further subdivided into the following blocks:

Categories	Section Titles
A00–A09	Intestinal infectious diseases
A15–A19	Tuberculosis
A20–A28	Certain zoonotic bacterial diseases
A30–A49	Other bacterial diseases
A50–A64	Infections with a predominantly sexual mode of transmission
A65–A69	Other spirochetal diseases
A70–A74	Other diseases caused by chlamydiae
A75–A79	Rickettsioses
A80–A89	Viral and prion infections of the central nervous system
A90–A99	Arthropod-borne viral fevers and viral hemorrhagic fevers
B00–B09	Viral infections characterized by skin and mucous membrane lesions

B10	Other human herpesviruses
B15–B19	Viral hepatitis
B20	Human immunodeficiency virus [HIV] disease
B25–B34	Other viral diseases
B35–B49	Mycoses
B50–B64	Protozoal diseases
B65–B83	Helminthiases
B85–B89	Pediculosis, acariasis, and other infestations
B90–B94	Sequelae of infectious and parasitic diseases
B95–B97	Bacterial and viral infectious agents
B99	Other infectious diseases

In coding infectious and parasitic diseases, the entire health record must be reviewed to identify

- Body site: for example, intestine, kidney, or blood
- Severity of the disease: for example, acute versus chronic
- Specific organism: for example, *Candida*, bacteria, virus, or parasite
- Etiology of infection: for example, food poisoning
- Associated signs, symptoms, or manifestations: for example, gangrene, bleeding, or Kaposi's sarcoma

Infectious and parasitic conditions can be classified in the following ways; thus, the coder should carefully review the Alphabetic Index. Remember that the primary axis for conditions in this chapter is the responsible organism. When coding, remember the following points:

- Use a single code to indicate the organism.
- Use combination codes to indicate both the organism and the condition.
- A dual classification is used for this chapter.

The coder is reminded that codes from Chapter 1 take precedence over codes from other chapters when coding the same condition. Also, be guided by the "Use additional code" notes in the Tabular List to assist with proper coding.

Laboratory Tests Used in the Diagnosis and Treatment of Infectious Diseases

Before reviewing specific categories in this chapter, it will be helpful to have a general understanding of some of the basic laboratory tests that can assist the physician in the diagnosis and treatment of infectious diseases.

Smear and Stain Examinations

The Gram stain technique is named for Dr. Christian Gram, who first described it in 1884. This technique can assist a physician in making a diagnosis by providing clues to identify the agent causing an infection, thus helping the physician determine the appropriate antibiotic to prescribe while waiting for culture results. Gram-positive organisms stain purple; Gram-negative organisms shed the stain and appear red. Some examples of Gram-positive and Gram-negative organisms include the following:

Gram-Positive Organisms	**Gram-Negative Organisms**
Staphylococcus	*Neisseria*
Streptococcus	*Branhamella (Moraxella)*

Anthrax   *Campylobacter*
Clostridium   *Enterobacteriaceae*
Lactobacillus   *Salmonella*
Actinomyces   *Klebsiella*
Listeria   *Yersinia*
Corynebacterium   *Morganella*
Peptococcus   *Vibrio*
Peptostreptococcus *Aeromonas*
                     Proteus
                     Serratia
                     Shigella
                     Citrobacter

When a good sputum specimen is obtained, the Gram stain is a rapid, simple, and inexpensive technique for diagnosing bacterial pneumonia.

In addition to separating bacteria into Gram-positive and Gram-negative groups, the Gram-staining process also indicates the shape of the bacterium. Bacteria may appear as rods or cocci. Examples of how the shape is used to classify bacteria include the following:

Shape	Organism
Cocci in chains	*Streptococci*
Cocci in clusters	*Staphylococci*
Straight rods	*Salmonella*
Brick-shaped rods	*Clostridium perfringens*

Acid-fast stains are used when bacteria do not stain easily with the Gram stain. Examples of acid-fast stains are Ziehl-Neelsen stain, Fluorochrome stain, and Kinyoun carbolfuchsin stain.

Other staining methods and the types of organisms that are examined by microscope include the following:

Name of Stain	Organism(s) Examined
Tzanck stain	Herpes simplex and varicella-zoster skin lesions
Silver stain	Treponema, fungi, *Pneumocystis carinii*, *Legionella*, rickettsiae
Periodic acid-Schiff	Fungi
Acridine orange	Bacteria, fungi, trichomonads
Methylene blue	Fecal leukocytes
Giemsa and Wright	Malaria, *Helicobacter pylori*

Cultures

In culturing specimens, the rate of growth, atmospheric needs (such as aerobic or anaerobic), and nutritional requirements of the bacterium are clues to its identification. Media commonly used in culturing are liquid (broths) and gel (agar). The grouping of bacterium growth on a culture is referred to as a colony. Additional clues for bacteria identification include odor, pigment production, and shape, size, and consistency of the colony.

Serologic Studies

Serologic studies are used to provide a specific diagnosis when attempts to identify an infectious agent are unsuccessful or impractical, or when culture techniques or facilities are unavailable. Often therapeutic decisions are made before the serologic test results can be made available.

Infectious diseases commonly diagnosed by serologic testing include syphilis, rubella, *Mycoplasma pneumoniae*, Lyme disease, and infectious mononucleosis.

Microorganisms That Cause Infections

Coders need to know the general categories of microorganisms that cause infections. Microorganisms that infect humans and induce disease include bacteria, parasites, fungi, and viruses. In terms of medicine, microbial diseases are classified according to the affected organ or system. For example, the bacterium *Staphylococcus aureus* can cause disease of the skin, bones, and respiratory tract. The Coxsackie virus B5 can induce symptoms involving the central nervous system, serous membranes, and skeletal and cardiac musculature. Remember that physicians and pathologists may use abbreviations for the various microorganisms.

Bacteria

Bacteria are one-celled, microscopic organisms that multiply by cell division. For millions of years, they were the dominant forms of life on earth. They are currently found in virtually all environments. Some bacteria are vital to the functioning of ecosystems; others cause infections and diseases in humans and animals.

Streptococcus pyogenes (group A) is an inhabitant of the upper respiratory tract and is spread by droplets or direct contact, especially in overcrowded conditions. When infection occurs in the upper respiratory tract, the result is acute exudative pharyngitis, with or without tonsillitis, peritonsillar abscess, or suppurative lymphadenitis. Other manifestations of *S. pyogenes* are impetigo, chronic renal failure, rheumatic fever, and carditis.

Streptococcus pneumoniae is a common organism found in the mouth of 10 to 40 percent of healthy people. Often referred to as pneumococcus, this organism causes lobar pneumonia in adults and sinusitis and otitis media in children. Pneumococcus also is the most common cause of meningitis in the elderly. A vaccine is available for these high-risk people. Other organisms include group D streptococcus, which sometimes is seen in patients with gastrointestinal neoplasms, and group G streptococcus, which causes a variety of infections, including bursitis, pleuropulmonary infections, and skin and soft-tissue infections.

S. aureus organisms may cause infections involving the skin and subcutaneous tissues, the eye, or the ear. These organisms also cause diseases such as pneumonia, endocarditis, osteomyelitis, food poisoning, and toxic shock syndrome. This organism can be transmitted by direct spread or through the bloodstream.

Clostridium difficile normally inhabits the bowel. In recent years, it has been recognized as a cause of pseudomembranous colitis. Diarrhea and fever are symptoms of intestinal infection caused by this organism.

Mycoplasma is a genus of bacteria, of which the three most common species that produce disease in humans are *M. pneumoniae*, *Mycoplasma hominis*, and *Ureaplasma urealyticum*. The latter two organisms are together referred to as genital mycoplasmas because of their connection with the genital tract. *M. pneumoniae* can cause other respiratory diseases, such as pneumonia, pharyngitis, laryngitis, bronchiolitis, and bronchitis.

Enterobacteriaceae is a large group of bacteria characterized by the shape of gram-negative rods. Infections that primarily affect the gastrointestinal tract are caused by the bacterium *Escherichia coli*.

Bacillus includes many bacteria, but only a few cause disease in humans. *Bacillus anthracis* and *Bacillus cereus* are causes of anthrax and food poisoning, respectively.

C. perfringens is an organism that normally inhabits the human intestines. This organism can cause cellulitis and food poisoning.

Chlamydia trachomatis bacteria cause an infection that affects the conjunctiva, urethra, and cervical canal. Conjunctival infections are spread by contaminated hands. A neonate born to an infected mother may contract an infection by passing through the infected birth canal. *C. trachomatis* infections in the genitals are spread by sexual contact.

Table 2.1 describes the locations of infections caused by common pathogens.

Parasites

A parasite is an organism that lives in or on another living organism. The Sporozoea is a class of microscopic parasites that can cause many human and animal diseases, including malaria. Worms also are classified as parasites, including the tapeworm, fluke, roundworm, pinworm, hookworm, and whipworm.

Table 2.1. Infection sites with common pathogens

Location of Infection	Common Pathogen
Urinary tract infections	*E. coli*, Klebsiella, Proteus, Pseudomonas sp., Enterococci

Intravenous catheter phlebitis or sepsis:
   Peripheral catheter
   Hyperalimentation line
	S. aureus, S. epidermidis, Klebsiella, Enterobacter, Pseudomonas sp., Candida sp., *S. epidermidis*, Enterococci

Arteriovenous shunt	*S. aureus, S. epidermidis*
Septic bursitis	*S. aureus*
Septic arthritis	*S. aureus*, gram-negative organisms in high-risk patients,* *H. influenzae* in children, Group B streptococci in neonates
Biliary tract	*E. coli*, Klebsiella sp., Enterococci, *B. fragilis* in elderly patients
Intra-abdominal abscess, peritonitis	*E. coli, B. fragilis*, Klebsiella sp., Enterococci
Burn wounds	Early: *S. aureus*, Streptococci Later: Gram-negative bacilli, fungi
Cellulitis, wound, and soft-tissue infections or large bowel perforation	*S. aureus*, Streptococci, Clostridium sp.
Pelvic abscess, postabortion or postpartum	Anaerobic streptococci, *B. fragilis*, Clostridium sp., *E. coli*, Enterococci
Acute osteomyelitis	*S. aureus, H. influenzae* in children, Group B streptococci in neonates, gram-negative organisms in high-risk patients*
*High-risk patients include the elderly, intravenous drug abusers, diabetics, and debilitated or immunocompromised patients.	

Fungi

Fungi also can cause infectious diseases, including poisonings, allergies, cutaneous or mucous membrane infections, and subcutaneous and invasive infections. However, most fungal infections do not spread from person to person.

One fungal infection, candidiasis infection, is so common that the disease has received several other names, such as moniliasis, thrush, and mycotic vulvovaginitis. The *Candida albicans* species causes this fungus disease. The disease may be localized to the mouth, throat, skin, scalp, vagina, fingers, nails, bronchi, lungs, or gastrointestinal (GI) tract.

The following conditions can lead to opportunistic infection by the pathogen *Candida*:

- Extreme youth (thrush or diaper rash)
- Physiologic change (pregnancy with vaginitis, postsurgical status)
- Administration of steroids
- Prolonged administration of antibiotics
- General debility (diabetes, malignancy, acquired immunodeficiency syndrome [AIDS])

Viruses

A virus is a minute, infectious microorganism that is much smaller than a bacterium and replicates only within a living host cell.

The following is a list of commonly known viral infections:

Adenoviridae (adenoviruses)
Arbovirus (encephalitis)
Aseptic meningitis
Cytomegalovirus (CMV)
Epstein-Barr virus
Hepatitis viruses
Herpes simplex virus
Human immunodeficiency virus
Influenza virus types A and B
Measles
Mumps
Papilloma viruses
Paralytic poliomyelitis
Respiratory syncytial virus
Rubella
Varicella zoster
Rabies

More information on common viral infections is presented later in this chapter.

In coding infectious and parasitic diseases, the entire health record must be reviewed to identify the following:

- Body site (such as lungs, liver, skin, or vagina)
- Severity of the disease (acute versus chronic)
- Specific organism or parasite (such as *Candida*, bacteria, or virus)
- Etiology of the infection (such as food poisoning)
- Associated signs, symptoms, or manifestations (such as jaundice or Kaposi's sarcoma)

Combination Codes and Multiple Coding

Chapter 1 of the ICD-10-CM code book includes many combination codes to identify both the condition and the causative organism; therefore, multiple coding is often necessary to completely describe an infectious condition or disease.

When coding infections, the Alphabetic Index should be checked very carefully for organism verus other subterm or site.

Drug-Resistant Infections

Two organisms identified in category Z22 that occur frequently in patients are methicillin resistant *Staphylococcus aureus* (MRSA) (code Z22.322) and methicillin susceptible *Staphylococcus aureus* (MSSA) (code Z22.321.) When a patient is diagnosed with an infection that is due to MRSA, and that infection has a combination code that includes the causal organism (such as septicemia or pneumonia due to *Staphylococcus aureus*), the appropriate combination code for that infection and its causal organism is assigned. The codes Z22.322 or Z22.321 are not assigned as additional codes, unless the physician specifically documents an infection that has become drug resistant.

When there is documentation of a current infection, such as a wound infection, that is due to MRSA or MSSA, and that infection does not have a combination code that includes the causal organism, the appropriate code to identify the infection or condition is assigned, with an additional code for MRSA (A49.02) or MSSA (A49.01). The coder would not assign a code from subcategory Z16.11, Resistance to penicillins, as an additional code.

The term *colonization* means that MRSA or MSSA is present on or in the body without necessarily causing illness. A positive colonization test may be documented as a "positive MRSA screen" or "positive MSSA screen." Either code Z22,322, Carrier or suspected carrier, methicillin resistant *Staphylococcus aureus* (MRSA) colonization, or Z22.321, Carrier or suspected carrier, methicillin methicillin-susceptible *Staphylococcus aureus* (MSSA) colonization, is assigned to identify the colonization or carrier status of the patient.

If a patient has both MRSA colonization and infection during an episode of care, code Z22.322,—Carrier or suspected carrier, methicillin resistant *Staphylococcus aureus* (MRSA) colonization—and a code for the MRSA infection may both be assigned.

Common Infectious Diseases

This section looks at various infectious diseases for which codes may need to be assigned. Each disease is described along with the coding used to report it.

Tuberculosis

Tuberculosis (A15–A19) is an acute or chronic infection caused by *Mycobacterium tuberculosis* and *Mycobacterium bovis*. Infection commonly occurs in the lungs, although it can occur in other sites, such as the meninges. In the primary infection of pulmonary tuberculosis, symptoms include fatigue, weakness, anorexia, weight loss, night sweats, and low-grade fever. Secondary infections are characterized by productive cough, hemoptysis, chest pain, and anorexia.

The diagnostic workup for tuberculosis includes the following:

- Purified protein derivative (PPD)
- Sputum culture (results may take three to six weeks)
- Acid-fast bacilli of sputum
- Chest x-ray

The fourth-character subclassification for use with categories A15–A10 identifies the various body systems or organs involved. Nonspecific reaction to tuberculin skin test without documentation of active tuberculosis is reported with code R76.11. A positive PPD is also classified to R76.11.

Streptococcal Sore Throat

Streptococcal sore throat (strep throat) is defined as an infection of the throat due to ß-hemolytic streptococci. It is characterized by a sudden onset of fever, malaise, headache, and nausea. The throat appears edematous and red, and exudate may or may not be present. When such symptoms are present, a throat culture is indicated. ICD-9-CM classifies strep throat to code J02.0. No additional code is necessary to identify the organism *(Streptococcus)* because it is already included in the title of code J02.0.

Septicemia and Sepsis

ICD-10-CM classifies septicemia by the underlying organism or systemic infection involved. A diagnosis of sepsis can neither be assumed nor ruled out on the basis of lab values alone. A code for sepsis can be assigned only when the physician makes such a diagnosis.

The terms *septic shock, severe sepsis, and sepsis* have been used interchangeably by physicians, but they are clinically distinct conditions and are no longer considered synonymous terms. ICD-10-CM is consistently updated to reflect current medical terminology regarding septic shock, sepsis, and septicemia.

Bacteremia (R78.81) is defined as the presence of bacteria in the bloodstream after trauma or a mild infection. The systemic inflammatory response syndrome (SIRS) is the systemic response to infection, trauma, burns, or other insult (for example, cancer) with symptoms that include fever, tachycardia, tachypnea, and leukocytosis. Severe sepsis (R65.2-) is defined as sepsis with associated acute or multiple organ dysfunction. Subcategory R65.2 is subdivided to identify whether it is associated with septic shock (R65.21) or occurs without septic shock (R65.20). Septic shock generally refers to circulatory failure associated with severe sepsis and therefore represents a type of acute organ dysfunction. The physician needs to specifically record "septic shock" in the diagnostic statement in order to code it as such.

Coding and Sequencing Rules for Sepsis and Severe and Septic Shock

The rules for coding and sequencing rules for sepsis and severe or septic shock are explained below.

Sepsis: With a diagnosis of sepsis, assign

- Appropriate code for the underlying systemic infection
- Assign code A41.9, Sepsis, unspecified organism, if the infection or causal organism is not listed

Because urosepsis is a nonspecific term, it should not be considered synonymous with sepsis. The physician should be queried if this term is used.

Severe Sepsis: When coding severe sepsis, a minimum of two codes are required:

- First, sequence a code for the underlying systemic infection followed by a code from subcategory R65.2, Severe sepsis. If documentation does not indicate the causal organism, assign code A41.9, Sepsis, unspecified organism, for the infection code.
- Assign an additional code for any associated organ dysfunction.

Septic Shock: This usually refers to circulatory failure that is associated with severe sepsis and subsequently represents a type of acute organ dysfunction. The following rules for coding should be observed:

- First, sequence the code for the systemic infection.
- Next, use code R65.21, Severe sepsis with septic shock, or code T81.12, Postprocedural septic shock.
- Additional codes for the other acute organ dysfunction should be assigned.

Sepsis and Severe Sepsis with a Localized Infection: If the reason for the encounter is both sepsis (or severe sepsis) and a localized infection (for example, pneumonia, cellulitis), code as follows:

- Code the underlying systemic infection first.
- Assign a secondary code for the localized infection.
- Code R65.2- is assigned as a secondary code if the patient has severe sepsis.

Sepsis Due to a Postprocedural Infection: In order to use a postprocedural infection code, the provider needs to document the relationship between the infection and the procedure. For such cases,

- First, assign the postprocedural infection code T80.2, Infections following infusion, transfusion, and therapeutic injection; T81.4, Infection following a procedure; T88.0, Infection following immunization; or O86.0, Infection of obstetric surgical wound.
- Code R65.2- should be assigned if the patient has severe sepsis.
- Finally, code any acute organ dysfunction if present.

Sepsis and Severe Sepsis Associated with a Noninfectious Condition or Process: Sometimes a condition or noninfectious process (for example, trauma) can ultimately lead to an infection resulting in sepsis or severe sepsis. In order to code this,

- Assign a code for the noninfectious condition first.
- The resulting infection is coded next.
- Assign code R65.2- if severe sepsis is present.
- Finally, code an associated organ dysfunction.

Meningitis

Bacterial meningitis (G00.9) is an inflammation of the meninges, a trio of membranes that surround the spinal cord and brain. Signs of infection are fever, chills, and malaise, increased cranial pressure exhibited as headache, and vomiting. Meningococcal meningitis is coded with A39.0.

Childhood Communicable Diseases

Chickenpox (B01.9), or varicella, is a common acute and highly contagious infection caused by the herpes virus varicella-zoster. Category B01 is further subdivided to identify the presence or absence of complications.

Measles (B05.9) is one of the most common illnesses known. Symptoms present with fever, followed by a rash. The subcategory is further subdivided to identify the presence or absence of complications.

Rubella (B06.9), or German measles, is an acute, mildly contagious viral disease that produces a rash for approximately three days, along with lymphadenopathy. It is transmitted through contact with blood, urine, stools, or nasopharyngeal secretions. This subcategory is further subdivided to identify complications. When rubella is documented as congenital (present at birth), code P35.0 should be assigned.

Herpes

Herpes zoster (B02.9), or shingles, is a severe infection caused by the varicella-zoster virus. It is characterized by painful skin blisters that follow the posterior roots of the spinal nerves or the fifth cranial nerve.

Herpes simplex (B00.9) is a recurrent viral infection caused by herpes virus hominis. Herpes type I is transmitted by oral and respiratory secretions and affects skin and mucous membranes. It commonly produces fever blisters and cold sores. Herpes type II affects primarily the genital area and is transmitted by sexual contact. Subcategory code B00.9 is further subdivided to identify specific complications. When herpes simplex is congenital (present at birth), code P35.2 should be assigned.

Viral Hepatitis

Viral hepatitis (B19.9) is an inflammation of the liver caused by a virus. Signs and symptoms of hepatitis include jaundice, nausea, aversion to smoking, and abdominal pain on liver palpitation. Serum levels such as SGOT, SGPT, and serum bilirubin will be elevated. The five forms of hepatitis include the following:

- **Type A (HAV)**: Highly contagious and usually transmitted by a fecal-oral route.
- **Type B (HBV)**: Transmitted by direct exchange of contaminated blood, human secretions, and feces.
- **Type C (HCV)**: Usually transmitted through transfused blood from asymptomatic donors.
- **Type D (HDV-delta)**: Found only in patients with an acute or chronic episode of hepatitis B.
- **Type E (HEV)**: Transmitted enterally.

Subcategories B15–B19 are further subdivided to identify whether or not hepatic coma is present.

Candidiasis

Candidiasis (B37.9) is a fungal infection caused by the genus *Candida*, especially *C. albicans*. Candidiasis is synonymous with moniliasis. It usually is a mild, superficial fungal infection commonly occurring in the nails, skin, mucous membranes, vagina, esophagus, and GI tract. Occasionally, the fungi can enter the bloodstream and invade major organs such as the kidneys, lungs, or brain. Subcategory B37.9 is further subdivided to identify the specific site affected.

Sexually Transmitted Diseases

Sexually transmitted diseases (STDs), or venereal diseases, are contagious conditions usually spread through sexual intercourse or genital contact. Syphilis is classified to subcategory A53.9, which includes types specified as congenital, juvenile, latent, or symptomatic (those affecting specific body systems, such as the cardiovascular or neurologic systems). Gonorrhea is classified to subcategory A54.9.

Infectious Gastroenteritis

Infectious gastroenteritis can be caused by a variety of organisms, including bacteria, viruses, and parasites. It is characterized by severe nausea, vomiting, anorexia, abdominal cramps, fever, malaise, muscular aches, prostration, hypokalemia, acidosis, metabolic alkalosis, and hyponatremia.

Several categories exist within ICD-10-CM to classify infectious gastroenteritis, including the following:

- Code A02.0, *Salmonella gastroenteritis*, which includes *Salmonella* food poisoning with gastroenteritis (*Salmonella* food poisoning not further specified as with gastroenteritis is reported with code A02.9).
- Subcategory A05.9, Other food poisoning (bacterial), which is further subdivided to identify specific organisms or types.

AIDS and Other HIV Infections

Code B20 is used for all types of HIV infections and also includes the following terms:

- Acquired immune deficiency syndrome [AIDS]
- AIDS-related complex [ARC]
- HIV infection, symptomatic

Code only confirmed cases of HIV infection. Remember that confirmation does not require positive serology or culture. The physician's statement that the patient is HIV positive or has an HIV-related illness is all that is needed.

Sequencing of HIV Codes

When a patient is seen for an HIV-related condition, the first-listed diagnosis is code B20, Human immunodeficiency virus. Any related HIV-related conditions should be coded next. When an HIV patient is seen for an unrelated condition (for example, injury), that condition is the first listed code followed by code B20 and then any additional diagnosis codes for any HIV-related conditions.

Additional codes that may be used on symptomatic or asymptomatic patients are listed as follows:

- Z21, Asymptomatic human immunodeficiency virus [HIV] infection status, is used when the test result is positive but the patient does not have any symptoms or complications and no established diagnosis of HIV infection.
- Code R75, Inconclusive laboratory evidence of HIV, is used when patients have inconclusive serology and no definitive diagnosis or manifestations of the disease.
- Code Z11.4, Encounter for screening for HIV, is when the patient is being seen to evaluate his or her HIV status. An additional code for any associated high-risk behavior can also be used (code Z72.89, Other problems related to lifestyle).
- Code Z71.7, HIV counseling, can be coded if any counseling is provided to the patient during an encounter for testing.
- Code Z20.6, Contact with and (suspected) exposure to HIV, is used when a patient has been exposed to HIV but has no signs or symptoms and has not been diagnosed with an HIV condition.
- Code R75 is used when the test results are inconclusive for HIV.

Sequelae of Infectious and Parasitic Diseases

Chapter 1 has four categories that can be used when there is a residual condition due to a previous infection or parasitic infestation:

- B90   Sequelae of tuberculosis
- B91   Sequelae of poliomyelitis
- B92   Sequelae of leprosy
- B94   Sequelae of other and unspecified infectious and parasitic diseases

Remember that the code for the residual is listed first followed by the sequelae code, unless indicated otherwise by the Alphabetic Index.

Chapter 2: ICD-10-CM Exercises

Review the following statements and cases and assign the appropriate codes:

1. AIDS with Kaposi's sarcoma of skin of lower leg

2. Toxic shock syndrome due to group A *Streptococcus*

3. Aseptic meningitis

Continued

4. Osteitis due to yaws

5. Measles with no complications

6. Gastroenteritis due to *Salmonella*

7. Rotavirus enteritis

8. Asymptomatic HIV infection

9. Staphylococcal sepsis

10. Acute poliomyelitis

11. Left dominant lower limb paralysis; late effect of poliomyelitis

12. Candidiasis infection of the mouth

13. Tinea pedis

14. Anthrax pneumonia

15. Encephalitis due to smallpox inoculation

16. Acute necrotizing otitis media in measles

17. Patient has brain damage resulting from previous viral encephalitis (two years ago).

18. Patient is seen for infectious gammaherpesviral mononucleosis with hepatomegaly.

19. This child is being seen for postmeasles otitis media.

20. Chronic moniliasis of vagina

21. Tuberculous calcifications of adrenal gland

22. Exposure to human immunodeficiency virus (HIV)

23. Inconclusive HIV test

24. Patient was diagnosed with acute respiratory distress due to Sin Nombre virus.

25. Patient has been diagnosed with herpes zoster of the conjunctiva.

Chapter 2: ICD-10-CM Exercises (continued)

26. Tuberculosis of tracheobronchial lymph nodes

27. *Clostridium difficile* (c. diff) colitis. This organism was resistant to multiple drugs.

28. Chronic gonococcal urethritis

29. Pelvic inflammatory disease as the result of sexually transmitted chlamydia

30. Latent syphilis of central nervous system

31. Measles complicated by otitis media

32. Gram-negative severe sepsis with acute respiratory failure

Neoplasms

Chapter 3

OBJECTIVES

After completing this lesson, you should be able to do the following:

- Apply knowledge of current, approved ICD-10-CM coding guidelines to assign and sequence accurate codes for diagnoses related to neoplasms
- Understand the definitions that describe the behavior of neoplasms
- Discuss the use and construction of morphology (M) codes
- Understand how to use the Neoplasm Table in the Alphabetic Index to Diseases
- Know how to correctly code neoplasms that are described as metastatic

ICD-10-CM

The term *neoplasm* refers to any new or abnormal growth. Chapter 2 in the ICD-10-CM code book classifies all neoplasms. Generally, these conditions are treated by referral to an oncologist. The following categories and section titles are included:

Categories	Section Titles
C00–C14	Malignant neoplasms of lip, oral cavity, and pharynx
C15–C26	Malignant neoplasms of digestive organs
C30–C39	Malignant neoplasms of respiratory and intrathoracic organs
C40–C41	Malignant neoplasms of bone and articular cartilage
C43–C44	Melanoma and other malignant neoplasms of skin
C45–C49	Malignant neoplasms of mesothelioma and soft tissue
C50	Malignant neoplasms of breast
C51–C58	Malignant neoplasms of female genital organs
C60–C63	Malignant neoplasms of male genital organs
C64–C68	Malignant neoplasms of urinary tract
C69–C72	Malignant neoplasms of eye, brain, and other parts of central nervous system
C73–C75	Malignant neoplasms of thyroid and other endocrine glands
C7A	Malignant neuroendocrine tumors

C7B	Secondary neuroendocrine tumors
C76–C80	Malignant neoplasms of ill-defined, other, secondary and unspecified sites
C81–C96	Malignant neoplasms of lymphoid, hematopoietic, and related tissue
D00–D09	In situ neoplasms
D10–D36	Benign neoplasms, except benign neuroendocrine tumors
D3A	Benign neuroendocrine tumors
D37–D48	Neoplasms of uncertain behavior, polycythemia vera, and myelodysplastic syndromes
D49	Neoplasms of unspecified behavior

In ICD-10-CM, the first axis for coding neoplasms is behavior, and the second axis is the anatomical site.

Behavior of Neoplasms

Definitions that describe the behavior of neoplasms include

- **Malignant:** Malignant neoplasms are collectively referred to as cancers. A malignant neoplasm can invade and destroy adjacent structures, as well as spread to distant sites to cause death.
- **Primary:** A primary site is the site where a neoplasm originated.
- **Secondary:** A secondary site is the site(s) to which the neoplasm has spread via:
  - ▸ Direct extension, in which the primary neoplasm infiltrates and invades adjacent structures
  - ▸ Metastasis to local lymph vessels by tumor cell infiltration
  - ▸ Invasion of local blood vessels
  - ▸ Implantation in which tumor cells shed into body cavities
- **In situ:** In an in situ neoplasm, the tumor cells undergo malignant changes but are still confined to the point of origin without invasion of surrounding normal tissue. The following terms also describe in situ malignancies:
  - ▸ Noninfiltrating
  - ▸ Noninvasive
  - ▸ Intraepithelial
  - ▸ Preinvasive carcinoma
- **Benign:** In benign neoplasms, growth does not invade adjacent structures or spread to distant sites but may displace or exert pressure on adjacent structures.
- **Uncertain behavior:** Neoplasms of uncertain behavior are tumors that a pathologist cannot determine to be either benign or malignant, because features of both are present.
- **Unspecified nature:** Neoplasms of unspecified nature include tumors in which neither behavior nor the morphology is specified in the diagnosis.

Neuroendocrine Tumors

Neuroendocrine tumors arise from endocrine or neuroendocrine cells that are scattered throughout the body, with the most common sites being the bronchi, stomach, small intestine, appendix, and rectum. Neuroendocrine tumors are usually classified according to the presumed embryonic site of origin, for example, the foregut (bronchi and stomach), midgut (small intestine and appendix), and hindgut (colon and rectum).

Neoplasm Table

The Alphabetic Index contains a table, the Neoplasm Table, which is indexed under the main term *neoplasm*.

The Neoplasm Table contains seven columns. The first column lists the anatomical sites in alphabetical order. The next six columns identify the behavior of the neoplasm. The first three of these six columns include codes for malignant neoplasms and are further classified as primary, secondary, and carcinoma (Ca) in situ. The fourth column identifies codes for benign neoplasms. The last two columns include codes for neoplasms of uncertain behavior and of unspecified type.

When many sites are indented under a main term, the listing for that term may run several pages long. Accurate coding requires the coder to search through all the subterms under the main heading.

Unspecified Lesion or Mass

When only the terms *lesion* or *mass* are documented in the record, the coder should refer to the Alphabetic Index's main terms mass or lesion and not select a code from the Unspecified Behavior column of the Neoplasm Table. If there is a diagnosis of "lump" with no index entry for the organ or site affected, check for information under mass. The main term *disease* may also be referenced if no specific site can be found under the term mass.

Instructions in the Alphabetic Index for Coding Neoplasms

The main terms and subentries in the Alphabetic Index assist the coder in locating the morphologic type of neoplasms. When a specific code or site is not listed in the index, cross-references direct the coder to the Neoplasm Table. The following steps should be followed in coding neoplasms:

1. Locate the morphology of the tumor in the Alphabetic Index. In most cases, the coder is directed to the Neoplasm Table. In other cases, the coder is provided with a code under the morphology type. For example:

Adenocarcinoma of the colon
> **Adenocarcinoma**—*see also* Neoplasm, malignant, by site

Acute lymphocytic leukemia
> **Leukemia, leukemic C95.9-**
>> lymphoid C91.9-

---

2. Follow the instructions under the main term in the Alphabetic Index. Instructions in the Alphabetic Index should be followed when determining which column to use in the Neoplasm Table. For example:

Adenomyoma (*see also* Neoplasm, by site, benign)

EXAMPLE: Malignant adenoma of colon

C18.9, Malignant neoplasm of colon, unspecified

Although the Alphabetic Index says to "*see also* Neoplasm, by site, benign," after the main term, *adenoma*, the coder is directed by the subterm, malignant, malignum, to "*see* Neoplasm, malignant, by site."

3. When a diagnostic statement indicates which column of the Neoplasm Table to reference but does not identify the specific type of tumor, the Neoplasm Table should be consulted directly.

EXAMPLE: Carcinoma in situ of cervix

D06.9, Carcinoma in situ of cervix, unspecified

After consulting the Neoplasm Table, code D06.9 from the *in situ* column is selected.

4. Any code numbers that are listed with a dash (C95.9-) require a fifth character to indicate that more numbers or letters are needed to complete the code.

5. Remember that all codes obtained from the Neoplasm Table should always be verified in the Tabular List.

Malignant Neoplasms

In ICD-10-CM, there are two basic types of malignant neoplasms:

- C00–C75, C76–C80   Solid
- C81–C96   Hematopoietic and lymphatic

Solid tumors are characterized by a single, localized point of origin and are considered as primary neoplasms of that site. These types of tumor are likely to spread to adjacent or remote sites (metastatic sites).

Unlike solid tumors, neoplasms of lymphatic and hematopoietic origin arise in the reticuloendothelial and lymphatic systems and blood-forming tissues. Characteristics of these types of tumors include:

- Originate in a single or multiple sites at the same time
- Instead of being confined to a single site, tumor cells generally circulate in the bloodstream and lymphatic system
- Spread to other sites in the hematopoietic and lymphatic system is not considered a secondary site but rather is still classified as a primary neoplasm

How to Code Solid Malignant Neoplasms

Solid malignant neoplasms can spread from the site of origin by direct extension or metastasis. Direct extension is when the tumor invades sites adjacent to the tumor, whereas metastasis involves the spread or invasion to distant sites. Clinicians use the terms *metastasis* and *secondary site* interchangeably.

Overlapping Sites

In some cases, the origin of the tumor (primary site) may involve two or more adjacent or contiguous sites. When this is the case, it is classified to subcategory .8, which refers to overlapping sites of the organ or site.

EXAMPLE: C02.8 Malignant neoplasm of overlapping sites of tongue

Multiple Malignancies

It is possible for a patient to have more than one malignant tumor in the same organ or site. When this occurs, the physician must determine whether this is a synchronous primary tumor or a metastatic or secondary site. Once this determination has been made by the physician, the sites can be properly coded as multiple primary sites or as a primary site with metastasis.

Coding Metastatic Sites

Metastatis sites can be coded in a variety of ways, depending on the specific diagnostic statement, as follows.

Metastatic "To" a Site

The terms *metastatic* and *metastasis* are used interchangeably for classifying a secondary malignant neoplasm in ICD-10-CM. Cancer described as "metastatic to a specific site" is interpreted as a secondary neoplasm of that site.

> **EXAMPLE:** Metastatic Carcinoma of the colon to the lung
>
> Primary Site: Colon
>
> Secondary Site: Lung

A code for the carcinoma of the colon is obtained from the Neoplasm Table using the Malignant Primary column. When coding the metastasis to the lung, again reference the Neoplasm Table, and obtain a code from the Malignant Secondary column.

A code for the primary neoplasm can be used as long as the neoplasm is still present (even if the patient is undergoing treatment such as radiotherapy or chemotherapy). Once the primary has been removed or eradicated, a history code from Category Z85, Personal history of malignant neoplasm, should be assigned. The fourth character under category Z85 indicates the body system where the neoplasm occurred. Any fifth and sixth characters specify the site or organ that is involved. The coder should reference the main term *History* in the Alphabetic Index to obtain the specific code needed. A family history of a malignancy can also be coded, and this code can also be located under the main term *History*.

Metastatic from a Site

Cancer described as metastatic "from" a site is interpreted as a primary neoplasm of that site.

> **EXAMPLE:** Metastatic carcinoma from the breast
>
> Primary Site: Breast
>
> Secondary Site: Code any metastatic site, if indicated

Remember that a code can be assigned from the Neoplasm Table for an unknown primary (C80.1), secondary (C79.9), in situ (D09.9), Benign (D36.9), Uncertain Behavior (D48.9), or Unspecified Behavior (D49.9) site. These codes can be located as the first entry in the Neoplasm Table immediately preceding the alphabetical listings of sites.

Multiple Metastatic Sites

When two or more sites are described as "metastatic" or "secondary," each site should be coded, and the codes are obtained from the Malignant Secondary column of the Neoplasm Table. If the primary site is still present and known, it should also be coded.

Metastasis of One Site

When only one site is stated in the diagnostic statement, and it is identified as "metastatic," the following steps should be taken:

1. In the Alphabetic Index, locate the morphological type of the neoplasm and then code to the primary condition of that site.

> **EXAMPLE:** Metastatic renal cell carcinoma of lung
>
> Primary Site: Kidney
>
> Secondary Site: Lung

When a specific site for the indicated morphology is not known, code as "unspecified site" for that anatomical site. The diagnosis would be coded as C34.90.

> **EXAMPLE:** Oat cell carcinoma
>
> The Alphabetic Index refers the coder to
>
> Carcinoma (main term in index)
>
> oat cell (subterm under main term in index)
>
> unspecified site C34.90

2. When the morphology type is not known or the only code that can be found is either C80.0 (Disseminated malignant neoplasm, unspecified) or C80.1 (Malignant [primary] neoplasm, unspecified), then the site described as metastatic in the diagnostic statement should be coded as primary malignant neoplasm, unless it is included in the following list of exceptions, in which case it must be coded as a secondary neoplasm of that site:

Bone	Brain
Diaphragm	Heart
Liver	Lymph nodes
Mediastinum	Meninges
Peritoneum	Pleura
Retroperitoneum	Spinal Cord
Sites classifiable to C76	

> **EXAMPLE:** A. Metastatic carcinoma of the bronchus
>
> Primary Site: Bronchus
>
> Secondary Site: Not specified (or unknown)
>
> B. Metastatic carcinoma of brain
>
> Primary Site: Unknown
>
> Secondary Site: Brain

Metastatic with No Site Stated

When the diagnostic statement does not list a specific site but the morphology type is known and qualified as metastatic, then the primary diagnosis is the morphological type. Also, list an additional code for a secondary neoplasm of unspecified site.

Coding Malignancies of Hematopoietic and Lymphatic Systems

Malignancies of hematopoietic and lymphatic systems are considered to be primary rather than secondary neoplasms.

Hodgkin's and Non-Hodgkin's Lymphoma

Hodgkin's lymphoma originates from lymphocytes, and the cancer is spread from one group of lymph nodes to another group. Under category C81, Hodgkin's lymphoma, the fourth characters specify the pathologic subtype, and fifth characters specify which lymph nodes are involved.

There are many types of non-Hodgkin's lymphoma, and these types can be fast or slow growing and can be formed from B-cells or T-cells. Category C82, Follicular lymphoma, provides a dual axis (grade and follicle description) classification to allow for the difference in terminology often seen in the patient's record. Fifth characters under this system identify the affected lymph nodes.

Leukemia

Leukemias are classified according to their type (lymphoid, myeloid, or monocytic) and their stage (acute or chronic). Fifth characters identify how the condition currently exists (without mention of having achieved remission, condition is in remission, or condition is in relapse).

Coding and Sequencing of Complications

Coding and sequencing of complications associated with the malignancies or with the therapy thereof are subject to the following guidelines:

- When an encounter is for the management of an anemia associated with the malignancy, and the treatment is only for the anemia, the appropriate anemia code is designated as the first-listed diagnosis and is followed by the appropriate code(s) for the malignancy. If a patient is admitted for treatment of malignancy and treated for anemia, the malignancy is sequenced as the principal diagnosis, and anemia is sequenced as an additional diagnosis.

- When an encounter is for management of an anemia associated with an adverse effect of radiotherapy, and the only treatment is for the anemia, the anemia is sequenced first, followed by code Y84.2, Radiological procedure, radiotherapy, as the cause of abnormal reaction of the patient, or of later complication, without mention of misadventure at the time of the procedure.

- When an encounter is for the management of dehydration due to the malignancy or the therapy, or a combination of both, and only the dehydration is being treated (intravenous rehydration), the dehydration is sequenced first, followed by the code(s) for the malignancy.

- When an encounter is for the management of a complication as a result of a surgical procedure, the first-listed diagnosis is the complication followed by the malignancy, which is coded as an additional diagnosis.

Chemotherapy, Immunotherapy, and Radiotherapy

- When surgical removal of a primary site malignancy is followed by chemotherapy, immunotherapy, or radiotherapy, the malignancy code is assigned as long as the chemotherapy, immunotherapy, or radiotherapy is actively administered. Even though the neoplasm has been removed surgically, the patient is still receiving therapy for that condition, and the active code for the malignant neoplasm must be assigned rather than a code describing history of carcinoma. After the therapy is complete, a code from Chapter 21 (Z codes) may be reported, rather than an active malignancy code.

- Encounters in which the patient receives chemotherapy, immunotherapy, or radiotherapy are sequenced as follows: When the encounter is solely for chemotherapy, code Z51.11, Encounter for antineoplastic chemotherapy, is sequenced first, followed by the appropriate ICD-10-CM code to identify the malignant neoplasm. When the encounter is solely for radiation therapy, code Z51.0, Encounter for antineoplastic radiation therapy, is sequenced first, followed by the appropriate ICD-10-CM code to identify the malignant neoplasm.

- ▸ When the encounter is for radium implant or insertion or for treatment by radioactive iodine, the code for the malignant neoplasm is reported, as this is not considered an admission for a radiotherapy session.
- ▸ When the encounter is only for antineoplastic immunotherapy, code Z51.12, Encounter for antineoplastic immunotherapy, is sequenced first, followed by the appropriate ICD-10-CM code to identify the malignant neoplasm.

Surgical Removal Followed by Recurrence

When a primary malignant neoplasm previously removed by surgery or eradicated by radiotherapy or chemotherapy recurs, the primary malignant code for that site is assigned, unless the Alphabetic Index directs otherwise.

Malignancy in a Transplanted Organ

Malignancy occurring in a transplanted organ should be coded as a transplant complication. The first-listed diagnosis should be code T86.-, Complications of transplanted organs and tissue, followed by the code C80.2, Malignant neoplasm associated with transplanted organ. In addition, a code for the specified malignancy can be added.

Follow-Up Examinations

Follow-up exams are routinely done to determine if there is any recurrence of the malignancy or any metastasis.

When there is no recurrence of a primary or secondary site, code as follows:

- Code Z08, Encounter for follow-up examination after completed treatment for malignant neoplasm, as the first-listed diagnosis
- An additional code to document the personal history of the malignant neoplasm (Z85.-)
- Code Z90.- can also be assigned for the acquired absence of an organ

When there is evidence of a primary recurrence, the malignancy code is the first-listed code. When there is evidence of recurrence of a secondary site, assign a neoplasm code for that site along with code Z85 to indicate personal history for the primary site.

Chapter 3: ICD-10-CM Exercises

Review the following statements and cases and assign the appropriate codes.

1. Glioma of the parietal lobe of the brain

2. Adenocarcinoma of prostate

3. Carcinoma in situ of vocal cord

4. Epidermoid carcinoma of the middle third of the esophagus

5. Galactorrhea due to pituitary adenoma

6. Benign melanoma of skin of right shoulder

7. Adrenal adenoma with primary hyperaldosteronism

8. Acute myeloid leukemia in remission

9. Hodgkin's granuloma of intra-abdominal lymph nodes and spleen

10. Recurrence of papillary carcinoma of bladder, low-grade transitional cell

11. Burkitt's lymphoma in multiple lymph nodes

12. Carcinoma of the brain from the lower lobe of the lungs

13. A 54-year-old woman was taken to the emergency department following episodes of shortness of breath and lethargy. She was treated mainly for her breathing difficulties. When a CT scan of the lungs was done to evaluate her breathing problem, it was noted that she had a mass in the right upper lobe of the lung. At that time, MRIs also were done of the bone, brain, and kidneys, all of which came back positive for metastatic deposits. A biopsy of the lung mass was done, and pathology was consistent with oat cell carcinoma. Radiation and chemotherapy were recommended.

    Discharge diagnosis: Oat cell carcinoma of the right upper lobe of the lung with metastasis to the bone (shoulder and hip), brainstem, and kidneys

    Code(s): _____

14. Inpatient encounter: An 87-year-old male was transferred from a local nursing home with complaints of partial hemiparesis. Immediately upon arrival, a CT scan of the brain was done that showed a mass in the left temporal lobe. The mass was biopsied and determined to be a glioblastoma. Radiation therapy was thought to be the best method of handling this tumor due to the patient's age and overall condition. He will return in a couple of weeks for his first treatment.

    Discharge diagnosis: Glioblastoma multiforme, left temporal lobe

    Code(s): _____

    Outpatient encounter: The elderly male patient was seen as an outpatient for administration of his first radiation treatment for glioblastoma multiforme, which was diagnosed only recently. Diagnosis: Radiotherapy for management of glioblastoma multiforme in the left temporal lobe

    Code(s): _____

15. A 53-year-old man was diagnosed with carcinoma of the lower portion of the esophagus one month ago. To date, he has received one chemotherapy treatment and, since the treatment, has been quite nauseated and not felt much like eating or drinking. He presents to the physician today for evaluation.

    Impression: Dehydration; carcinoma of the lower third of the esophagus

    Code(s): _____

16. Patient has been diagnosed with metastatic carcinoma of pancreas and omentum.

Continued

17. Multiple myeloma

18. Physician discusses with the patient her diagnosis of infiltrating papillary transitional cell carcinoma of the neck of the urinary bladder.

19. The patient is diagnosed with the following neoplasm: Hodgkin's sarcoma of thoracic lymph nodes.

20. Carcinoma in situ of right breast

21. Adenoma of the islet cells of the pancreas

22. Adenocarcinoma of rectum and anus

23. Aleukemic myeloid leukemia that is in remission

24. Multiple myeloma not having achieved remission

25. Not classified peripheral T-cell lymphoma of intrapelvic lymph nodes

26. Subacute monocytic leukemia in remission

27. Melanoma of the left breast and left arm

28. Lipomatous neoplasm (benign) of skin and subcutaneous tissue of right arm

29. Patient had left breast carcinoma four years ago, and a left mastectomy was performed. She has been well since that time with no further treatment except for yearly checkups. The patient is now being seen with visual disturbances, dizziness, headaches, and blurred vision. Workup was completed which revealed metastasis to the brain's accounting for these symptoms. This was identified as being metastatic from the breast, not a new primary.

30. Neoplasm of unspecified behavior of retina and choroid

Diseases of the Blood and Blood-Forming Organs

OBJECTIVES

After completing this lesson, you should be able to do the following:

- Apply knowledge of current, approved ICD-10-CM coding guidelines to assign and sequence accurate codes for diagnoses related to diseases of the blood and blood-forming organs, including hemorrhagic disorders and diseases of white blood cells
- Identify the various anemias and the coding guidelines for each type
- Discuss the three types of coagulation defects
- Discuss the various diseases of white blood cells

ICD-10-CM

Fluids constitute more than one half of an adult's weight under normal circumstances, and blood is one of the body's most important fluids. Blood is composed of a liquid called plasma, red blood cells (RBCs or erythrocytes), white blood cells (WBCs or leukocytes), and platelets. The study of blood and blood-forming tissues is called hematology, and the physician who studies blood is a hematologist.

Chapter 3 of the ICD-10-CM code book, Diseases of the blood and blood-forming organs, includes anemias, coagulation defects, purpura, and other hemorrhagic conditions and diseases of the white blood cells.

Chapter 3, Diseases of the blood and blood-forming organs and certain disorders involving the immune mechanism (D50–D89), includes the following blocks:

D50–D53	Nutritional anemias
D55–D59	Hemolytic anemias
D60–D64	Aplastic and other anemias and other bone marrow failure syndromes
D65–D69	Coagulation defects, purpura, and other hemorrhagic conditions
D70–D77	Other disorders of blood and blood-forming organs
D78	Intraoperative and postprocedural complications of spleen
D80–D89	Certain disorders involving the immune mechanism

Anemias

Anemia is characterized by a decrease in the number of erythrocytes, the quantity of hemoglobin, or the volume of packed red cells in the blood. Laboratory data reflect a decrease in RBCs, hemoglobin (Hgb), or hematocrit (Hct).

Deficiency Anemias

Codes used to describe deficiency anemias are included in categories D50–D53. The most common type—iron deficiency anemia (category D50)—is caused by an inadequate absorption or excessive loss of iron. Iron deficiency anemia due to chronic blood loss is reported with code D50.0. The underlying cause of the bleeding, such as an ulcer, menorrhagia, or cancer, also should be coded when documented in the health record. Without further specification, iron deficiency anemia is reported with code D50.9. Iron deficiency anemia due to acute blood loss (also known as acute posthemorrhagic anemia) is reported with code D62. It is defined as a normocytic, normochromic anemia developing as a result of rapid loss of large quantities of RBCs during bleeding. It may occur as a result of trauma with severe bleeding, rupture of an aneurysm, arterial erosion, cancerous or ulcerative lesions, and complications of surgery from excessive blood loss.

Category D51 describes other deficiency anemias, including

- D51.0 Pernicious anemia
- D51.3 Vitamin B12 deficiency anemia
- D52.0 Dietary folate deficiency anemia
- D53.0 Protein deficiency anemia
- D53.1 Other megaloblastic anemias, not elsewhere classified
- D53.8 Other specified nutritional anemias
- D53.9 Nutritional anemia, unspecified

Hemolytic Anemias

Hemolytic anemia refers to an abnormal reduction of RBCs caused by an increased rate of RBC destruction and the inability of the bone marrow to compensate. Hemolytic anemias may be hereditary (category D58) or acquired (category D59).

Hereditary Hemolytic Anemias

Hereditary hemolytic anemias are caused by intrinsic abnormalities involving structural defects of RBCs or defects of globin synthesis or structure. Categories D55–D58 include the following common hematologic disorders:

- D56 Thalassemia
- D57 Sickle-cell disorders
- D58 Other hereditary hemolytic anemias

Sickle-Cell Anemia

It is important to understand the difference between sickle-cell trait and sickle-cell disease. When a child receives the sickle-cell genetic trait from only one parent, he or she is considered a carrier of the trait (D57.3). When the child receives the trait from both parents, he or she has sickle-cell disease (D57.0-, D57.1, D57.2-, D57.4-, and D57.8-). When the physician documents both sickle-cell trait and sickle-cell disease, only the code for the disease is reported.

Acquired Hemolytic Anemias

Acquired hemolytic anemias are usually caused by extrinsic factors, such as infection, drugs or toxins, abnormal immune responses, and others. ICD-10-CM classifies acquired hemolytic anemia to category D59, with fourth characters to describe the specific type or cause. For example, code D59.0 identifies autoimmune hemolytic anemias.

Aplastic Anemia

Aplastic anemia is caused by an abnormal reduction of RBCs due to a lack of bone marrow production. The aplastic anemias include a diverse group of bone marrow disorders, most of which involve not just anemia but also pancytopenia. Half the aplastic anemia cases are attributed to exposure to a toxin, and half are determined to be of unknown causes. Toxins that can result in aplastic anemia include radiation and chemotherapy. ICD-10-CM classifies aplastic anemias to categories D60.- and D61.-, with fourth and fifth characters to indicate the specific type. For example, pancytopenia is reported with code D61.81-. Aplastic anemia without further specification is reported with code D61.9.

Acquired pure red cell aplasia is a form of aplastic anemia. Code D60.9, Red cell aplasia, may also be described as acquired red cell aplasia, unspecified.

Anemia Due to Blood Loss

The coder must clearly understand the difference between anemia due to acute blood loss as opposed to anemia due to chronic blood loss. Acute blood loss results from a significant and sudden blood loss over a short period of time. Acute blood loss may be due to trauma or rupture and can also occur following surgery. Acute blood loss following surgery is not necessarily a complication of any procedure and would not be coded as a postoperative complication unless the physician specifically states that it is. This type of blood loss may or may not result in anemia, and the coder should not assign such a code unless the physician documents the anemia. Chronic blood loss is a condition that occurs over a long period of time and often goes undetected. Listed are some codes that can be used in postoperative conditions:

- D64.9, Anemia, unspecified, is used as the default code when postoperative anemia is recorded without specification of acute blood loss.
- D62, Acute posthemorrhagic anemia, is assigned when postoperative anemia is due to blood loss.
- D50.0, Iron deficiency anemia secondary to blood loss (chronic), is coded when neither the diagnosis nor the review of the patient's record indicates whether the blood loss anemia is acute or chronic.

Coagulation Defects

Coagulation defects are disorders of the platelets resulting in serious bleeding due to a deficiency of one or more clotting factors. ICD-10-CM classifies coagulation defects, purpura, and other hemorrhagic conditions to D65–D69 with fourth and fifth characters that identify the specific type. Some common types of coagulation defects are recognized:

- **Hemophilia A (classic hemophilia)**—The most common type of coagulation defect (affects 1 in 5,000) and occurs as a result of factor VIII deficiency. It is inherited as an

X-linked recessive disorder that is transmitted by females and affects males. ICD-10-CM classifies classic hemophilia to category D66.

- **Hemophilia B (Christmas disease)**—Results from a deficiency of factor IX (affects 1 in 25,000). Like hemophilia A, this type is transmitted as an X-linked recessive trait. ICD-10-CM classifies hemophilia B to category D67.

- **Hemophilia C**—An autosomal recessive disease caused by a deficiency in factor XI. ICD-10-CM classifies this condition to code D68.1.

Other conditions are often confused with coagulation defects. For example, a patient being treated with Coumadin, heparin, or another anticoagulant may develop bleeding or a hemorrhage even if the anticoagulant is taken correctly. When this occurs, assign code T45.5-, Poisoning by, adverse effect of and underdosing of anticoagulants and antithrombotic drugs to indicate any administered anticoagulant, with code D68.32, Hemorrhage disorder due to extrinsic circulating anticoagulants. The code D68.31- would not be assigned unless the physician documents a hemorrhagic disorder due to intrinsic circulatory anticoagulants.

Another condition confused with coagulation defects is prolonged prothrombin time or other abnormal coagulation profiles without underlying disease. This condition is not coded as a coagulation defect. Code R79.1 is assigned to report an abnormal coagulation profile without disease.

Purpura and Other Hemorrhagic Conditions

Codes describing purpura and other hemorrhagic disorders are included in category D69. Thrombocytopenia is characterized by an abnormally low platelet count. Two types of thrombocytopenia are recognized: primary and secondary. Primary thrombocytopenia may be idiopathic, congenital, or hereditary, and is classified to code D69.49. Fourth characters designate specific types of primary thrombocytopenia. Secondary thrombocytopenia may result from drug use, massive blood transfusions, extracorporeal circulation of blood, malignancies, portal hypertension, damaged blood vessels, and infectious processes. ICD-10-CM classifies secondary thrombocytopenia to code D69.59. An additional code can be assigned to identify the drug or external cause. Subcategory code D69.5 excludes heparin-induced thrombocytopenia.

Diseases of the White Blood Cells

Categories D70–D77 classify diseases of the WBCs with fourth characters that identify the specific type of disorder. Two types of WBCs circulate in the body: granular and nongranular (agranular) leukocytes. Granular leukocytes include neutrophils, eosinophils, and basophils. Nongranular leukocytes include lymphocytes and monocytes. Agranulocytosis (also known as neutropenia) is an acute condition characterized by the absence of neutrophils or severe neutropenia and an extremely low granulocyte count. The most common cause is drug toxicity or hypersensitivity caused by large-dose and long-duration drugs. Neutropenia commonly occurs in patients receiving chemotherapy. ICD-10-CM classifies neutropenia to category D70. Fourth characters classify various types of neutropenia. A notation under this subcategory instructs the coder to "Use additional code for any associated fever (R50.81) or mucositis (J34.81, K12.3-, K92.81, N76.81)."

Additional subcategories and codes under D70-D77 designate other disorders of WBCs:

- D76.2   Hemophagocytic syndrome, infection associated
- D72.819   Decreased white blood cell count, unspecified
- D72.829   Elevated white blood cell count, unspecified

Disorders of the Immune System

Categories D80–D89 delineate various disorders of the immune system. Exceptions are those conditions due to or associated with HIV, as these are classified to code B20. The immune disorders include the following categories:

- D80 Immunodeficiency with predominantly antibody defects
- D81 Combined immunodeficiencies
- D82 Immunodeficiency associated with other major defects
- D83 Common variable immunodeficiency
- D84 Other immunodeficiencies
- D86 Sarcoidosis
- D89 Other disorders involving the immune mechanism, not elsewhere classified

Chapter 4: ICD-10-CM Exercises

Review the following statements and cases and assign the appropriate codes:

1. Iron deficiency anemia secondary to blood loss

2. Idiopathic primary thrombocytopenia

3. Familial polycythemia

4. Folate deficiency anemia due to dietary causes

5. Hereditary megaloblastic anemia

6. Screening for iron deficiency anemia

7. Inpatient admission: An 89-year-old man with heart palpitations and abdominal pain was brought by his daughter to see the physician. The physician ordered an EKG, a complete blood count (CBC), and an upper GI workup. The GI workup revealed significant gastritis. The EKG was not significantly abnormal. The CBC revealed the following: Hct: 25%; Hgb: 6.4; and WBC: 5,000. The cardiologist indicated that he believed the palpitations were a symptom of the patient's anemia. Social services were notified, because the physician attributed the anemia to nutritional deficiency. The patient received three units of packed cells and was discharged with a prescription for Tagamet.

    Discharge diagnoses: Anemia; gastritis

    Code(s):

8. A patient receives a blood transfusion for severe anemia due to her left breast carcinoma.

Continued

9. Congenital red cell aplastic anemia

10. A young adult is seen by her family physician complaining of extreme fatigue all the time. The physician questions the young lady about her eating habits and discovers that she eats mostly sweets and junk food. He orders blood work, and, after reviewing the results, diagnoses iron deficiency anemia due to inadequate dietary iron intake. How would this condition be coded?

11. A patient presents at the Walk-In Clinic and was diagnosed with idiopathic thrombocytopenia purpura. How should this be coded?

12. Anemia due to end-stage renal disease

13. Severe combined immunodeficiency [SCID] with low T- and B-cell numbers

14. Deficiency of factor I

Endocrine, Nutritional, and Metabolic Diseases

OBJECTIVES

After completing this lesson, you should be able to do the following:

- Apply knowledge of current ICD-10-CM coding guidelines to assign and sequence accurate codes for diagnoses related to endocrine, nutritional, and metabolic diseases
- Identify the types of diabetes mellitus and the complications and manifestations associated with the various types
- Delineate the major types of nutritional disorders and metabolic disorders

ICD-10-CM

Chapter 4 of the ICD-10-CM code book provides codes for endocrine, nutritional, and metabolic diseases. Typically, these types of disorders are treated by endocrinologists, allergists, immunologists, and physicians specializing in internal medicine or general practice.

The endocrine system involves glands that are located throughout the body. These glands secrete hormones into the bloodstream. Some of the major endocrine glands are the thyroid, adrenals, ovaries, and testicles. The best known of the endocrine disorders is diabetes mellitus (DM).

Chapter 4 is subdivided into the following sections:

Categories	Section Titles
E00–E07	Disorders of thyroid gland
E08–E13	Diabetes mellitus
E15–E16	Other disorders of glucose regulation and pancreatic internal secretion
E20–E35	Disorders of other endocrine glands
E36	Intraoperative complications of endocrine system
E40–E46	Malnutrition
E50–E64	Other nutritional deficiencies
E65–E68	Overweight, obesity, and other hyperalimentation
E70–E88	Metabolic disorders
E89	Postprocedural endocrine and metabolic complications and disorders, not elsewhere classified

Diabetes Mellitus

Diabetes mellitus is a metabolic disease in which insulin production by the pancreas is damaged or absent. DM may be due to both hereditary and nonhereditary factors, such as obesity, surgical removal of the pancreas, and the action of certain drugs. When the pancreas does not produce insulin, glucose (sugar) is not broken down so that it can be used and stored by the body cells. The result is too much sugar in the blood (hyperglycemia), which in turn spills into the urine (glycosuria). Saturation of the blood and urine with glucose draws water out of the body, causing dehydration and thirst. Other symptoms of DM include excessive hunger, marked weakness, and weight loss.

The following laboratory findings indicate a diagnosis of DM as per the American Diabetes Association:

In order to determine whether or not a patient has prediabetes or diabetes, healthcare providers conduct a fasting plasma glucose test (FPG) or an oral glucose tolerance test (OGTT). Either test can be used to diagnose prediabetes or diabetes. The American Diabetes Association recommends the FPG because it is easier, faster, and less expensive to perform.

With the FPG test, a fasting blood glucose level between 100 and 125 mg/dl signals prediabetes. A person with a fasting blood glucose level of 126 mg/dl or higher has diabetes.

In the OGTT test, a person's blood glucose level is measured after a fast and two hours after drinking a glucose-rich beverage. If the two-hour blood glucose level is between 140 and 199 mg/dl, the person tested has prediabetes. If the two-hour blood glucose level is at 200 mg/dl or higher, the person tested has diabetes.

DM affects 7.8 percent of the total United States population and is one of the leading causes of new cases of blindness. Many patients on dialysis have end-stage renal disease secondary to diabetic nephropathy. Many cases of lower extremity amputations take place in people with diabetes.

Treatment consists of insulin regulation by insulin injection, oral antidiabetic agents, or a controlled diet.

DM is classified into three major category types:

- Type 1
- Type 2
- Secondary (due to a drug or chemical or to an underlying condition)

The DM categories are listed as follows:

- E08   Diabetes mellitus, due to underlying conditions
- E09   Drug or chemical induced diabetes mellitus
- E10   Type 1 diabetes mellitus
- E11   Type 2 diabetes mellitus
- E13   Other specified diabetes mellitus

The type of diabetes is the essential element in code selection in one of the above-listed categories. If the type of diabetes is not stated or the patient's record is not clear, the default is always category E11 or Type 2. Remember that just because the patient may be receiving insulin, it does not mean that the type of diabetes is type 1.

Type 1 Diabetes Mellitus (E10)

Type 1 diabetes can also be described as

- Ketosis-prone
- Juvenile type

- Juvenile onset
- Juvenile diabetes

The patient's age is not the sole determining factor for type 1, but most type 1 patients develop the condition before reaching puberty. Type 1 diabetes is caused by the failure of the body to produce any insulin or by a decrease in insulin production. Therefore, patients require regular insulin injections to sustain life. Long term (current) use of insulin, code Z79.4, is actually not required to code type 1 diabetes, because these patients require insulin, and it should not be assigned to provide additional information.

Type 2 Diabetes Mellitus (E11)

Type 2 diabetes is also referred to as ketosis resistant. With this type of diabetes, insulin is produced but not in sufficient quantity or the body may not be able to utilize the insulin adequately. Type 2 diabetics can usually be maintained with diet and exercise or with hypoglycemic agents, thereby not usually requiring insulin. If a type 2 diabetic must use insulin for control, code Z79.4, Long-term (current) use of insulin, can be used if the insulin is given temporarily to regulate the patient's blood sugar.

Secondary Diabetes (E13.9)

Secondary diabetes is a condition caused by some other condition (E08) or event, such as drugs or chemicals (E09), an infection, or the result of therapy, such as removal of the pancreas. It may also be the result of an adverse effect of a correctly administered medication, or a poisoning or sequelae caused by medication.

Secondary diabetes can be coded as follows:

- E08   Secondary diabetes due to an underlying condition
- E09   Secondary diabetes due to a drug or chemical
- The Tabular List will indicate the proper sequencing of codes for categories E08 and E09
- Secondary diabetes due to a pancretectomy (E89.1, Postprocedural hypoinsulinemia) with an additional code from category E13. Acquired total absence (Z90.410) or acquired partial absence (Z90.411) of pancreas can also be coded.
- Code Z94.4 for long term use of insulin can also be used for those patients who routinely use insulin.

Complications and Manifestations

ICD-10-CM classifies DM to categories E08–E13, which are further subdivided to identify the presence or absence of complications or manifestations of the diabetes. When sequencing DM and the manifestation or complication, remember that the code used is based on the reason for the encounter. As many codes as needed should be assigned to identify all of the patient's conditions.

A number of acute metabolic complications may occur with DM:

- Hyperosmolarity with coma without nonketotic hyperglycemic-hyperosmolar coma
- Ketoacidosis with or without coma
- Hyperglycemia with or without coma

Diabetic patients are also susceptible to chronic conditions that can affect the renal, nervous, and peripheral vascular systems (for example, eyes and feet).

Diabetes with Renal Manifestations

Diabetic kidney complications are coded to E08-E13 with .21 for diabetic nephropathy, .22 for chronic kidney disease, and .29 for other kidney complications. Patients who have both diabetes and hypertension may also develop chronic kidney disease. When this is the case, three codes are required:

- One code for diabetes with a renal manifestation (E08–E13 with .22)
- Second code from either category I12 or I13 (hypertension codes)
- Third code from category N18 for the stage of the chronic kidney disease

Diabetes with Ophthalmic Manifestations

A true diabetic cataract, or snowflake cataract, is rare and should be assigned a code for diabetic cataract when the physician describes the condition as such. Senile (or age-related) cataracts in persons with DM are not classified as manifestations of the diabetes. Use a code from category H25, Age-related cataract, and a code from category E08–E13 to code senile cataracts in a diabetic patient.

Diabetes with Neurological Manifestations

Peripheral, cranial, or autonomic neuropathy are chronic manifestations of DM. Subclassifications for diabetic neurological complications are listed as follows:

- E08–E13 with .40, unspecified diabetic neuropathy
- E08–E13 with .41, diabetic mononeuropathy
- E08–E13 with .42, diabetic polyneuropathy
- E08–E13 with .43, diabetic autonomic (poly)neuropathy
- E08–E13 with .44, diabetic amyotrophy
- E08–E13 with .49, other diabetic neurological complications

Diabetes with Peripheral Circulatory Disorders

Arteriosclerosis occurs earlier and more extensively in diabetic than in nondiabetic patients. Coronary artery disease, cardiomyopathy, and cerebrovascular disease are not considered complications of DM, but a frequent complication of DM is peripheral vascular disease (with and without gangrene). DM, along with other circulatory complications, is coded to E08–E13 with .59.

Diabetes with Other Specified Manifestations

Other specified manifestations of DM would be classified to subcategory codes E08–E13 with .61-, .62-, or .63-. The coder is instructed to use an additional code to identify the manifestation, such as diabetic bone changes.

Diabetic Foot Ulcers

The underlying cause of foot ulcers in a diabetic patient may be diabetic neuropathy, peripheral vascular disease, or superimposed infection. In the latter case, ulcers are not coded as a diabetic complication; code the diabetes, the infection or causative organism (when applicable and when specified), and the specific site of the ulcer with sequencing, depending on circumstances of admission or encounter.

Organic Impotence

Organic impotence is often due to peripheral vascular disease or diabetic peripheral vascular disease. One should first code either E08–E13 with .40 or E08–E13 with .51. Also use code N52.1 for erectile dysfunction due to diseases classified elsewhere.

Complication Due to Insulin Pump Malfunction

Some diabetic patients need to use an insulin pump to receive their insulin therapy. Should the insulin pump fail, either underdosing or overdosing of insulin can occur, and this would be considered a mechanical complication. A code from subcategory T85.6—Mechanical complication of other specified internal and external prosthetic device, implants, and grafts—should be used to code this condition. The specific malfunction of the insulin pump may be a breakdown (T85.614), displacement (T85.624), or leakage (T85.633).

Diabetes Mellitus Complicating Pregnancy

Pregnant women who have diabetes should be assigned a code from category O24—DM in pregnancy, childbirth, and puerperium—first and then assign a code for the diabetes. If insulin is used on a long-term basis, code Z79.4 can also be assigned.

Gestational Diabetes

Sometimes during pregnancy, a condition of abnormal glucose tolerance, or gestational diabetes, will be found in a woman who is not a diabetic. Code O24.4, Gestational DM, is the code assigned on the basis of how the diabetes is controlled (diet or insulin) and whether the diabetes occurred in pregnancy, during childbirth, or during the puerperium. Code Z79.4 should not be used along with codes from subcategory O24.4. If a patient has an abnormal glucose tolerance during pregnancy but is never diagnosed with gestational diabetes, assign a code from subcategory O99.81, Abnormal glucose complicating pregnancy, childbirth and the puerperium.

Diabetes Mellitus in Newborns of a Diabetic Mother

When newborns are born to a diabetic mother, the baby may or may not be affected by the mother's diabetes. Codes are assigned in the following manner:

- Normal infant born to a diabetic mother, baby does not have diabetes or increased blood sugar, should be coded as:
    1. Z38.00   Single liveborn
    2. Z83.3   Family history of diabetes mellitus
    3. P00.89   Newborn (suspected to be) affected by other maternal condition

- Newborn has either a transient decrease in blood sugar or a transient hyperglycemia (P70.0, P70.1, P70.2, P70.3, or P70.4)

Remember that these codes can only be assigned if the maternal diabetes had an effect on the baby.

Hypoglycemia

Hypoglycemia is defined by a blood sugar level below 50 to 60 mg/dl. It can be caused by an imbalance in the amount of insulin taken, food eaten, or activity. Hypoglycemia can occur in patients both with and without diabetes. If the patient does not have diabetes, use code E15, Nondiabetic hypoglycemic coma. Category E15 also includes drug-induced insulin coma in a nondiabetic patient. For hypoglycemia, NOS, assign code E16.2. In a diabetic patient, hypoglycemia with coma is coded as E08–E13 with .641, or E08–E13 with .649 if there is no coma mentioned.

Nutritional Disorders

Categories E40–E64 classify nutritional disorders (for example, deficiency of specific vitamins and minerals). Several codes are necessary to identify overweight and obesity:

- E66.01 Morbid (severe) obesity due to excess calories
- E66.09 Other obesity due to excess calories
- E66.1   Drug-induced obesity
- E66.2   Morbid (severe) obesity with alveolar hypoventilation
- E66.3   Overweight
- E66.8   Other obesity
- E66.9   Obesity, unspecified

Category E66 requires the use of an additional code (Z68.-) to indicate the body mass index (BMI). It is a measure of weight for height and should be based on health record documentation.

Chapter 5: ICD-10-CM Exercises

Review the following statements and cases and assign the appropriate codes:

1. Moderate protein-calorie malnutrition

2. Vitamin B12 deficiency

3. Diabetic nephropathy

4. Familial combined hyperlipidemia

5. Polyuria, polydipsia; rule out diabetes mellitus (outpatient visit)

6. Cystic fibrosis

7. Wilson's disease

8. Graves' disease with thyrotoxic crisis

9. Pure hypercholesterolemia

10. Inappropriate antidiuretic hormone secretion syndrome

11. Acute infantile rickets

12. Juvenile hypopituitarism

13. Stein-Leventhal syndrome

14. Nutritional marasmus

15. Outpatient visit: A patient was evaluated for severe malnutrition and iron deficiency anemia secondary to her previously diagnosed amyotrophic lateral sclerosis. Social services were contacted for help with meals.

    Impression: Malnutrition, anemia; amyotrophic lateral sclerosis.

    Codes:

16. Hypoinsulinemia following total pancreatectomy

17. Progressive type 1 diabetic nephropathy with hypertensive renal disease and Stage 5 chronic kidney disease

18. Nonpressure chronic ulcer of unspecified heel with necrosis of bone. Patient also has diabetes, which physician states has caused this ulcer.

19. Diabetes mellitus, type 1, with acute osteomyelitis of great toe of right foot

20. Leakage of insulin pump causing patient to not receive the proper amount of insulin for her type 1 diabetes

21. Gestational diabetes occurring in pregnancy controlled by diet

22. Infantile hypoglycemia

23. Hemochromatosis due to repeated red blood cell transfusion

24. Congenital myxedema

25. Increased secretion of pancreatic growth hormone-releasing hormone

26. Morbid obesity with a BMI of 42 in an adult

27. Conn's syndrome

28. Familial hypocalciuric hypercalcemia

29. A 25-year-old male patient with type 1 diabetes mellitus, taking insulin is admitted because he is having symptoms of nausea, severe vomiting, increased frequency of urination, and polydipsia. The patient is also severely dehydrated. The patient was hydrated, and, as a result, his blood sugar decreased from more than 600 to normal levels. The patient was diagnosed with diabetic ketoacidosis, type 1.

30. Patient has steroid-induced diabetes mellitus due to the prolonged use of corticosteroids, which have been discontinued. The patient's diabetes is managed with insulin.

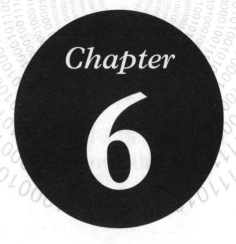

Chapter

6

Mental, Behavioral, and Neurodevelopmental Disorders

OBJECTIVES

After completing this lesson, you should be able to do the following:

- Apply knowledge of current ICD-10-CM coding guidelines to assign and sequence accurate codes for diagnoses related to mental disorders
- Identify the various types of mental disorders
- Differentiate between alcohol and alcoholism and drug abuse or drug dependence
- Determine the difference in types of affective disorders

ICD-10-CM

Chapter 5 of the ICD-10-CM code book classifies mental disorders into the following blocks:

Categories	Section Titles
F01–F09	Mental disorders due to known physiological conditions
F10–F19	Mental and behavioral disorders due to psychoactive substance use
F20–F29	Schizophrenia, schizotypal, delusional, and other nonmood psychotic disorders
F30–F39	Mood [affective] disorders
F40–F48	Anxiety, dissociative, stress-related, somatoform, and other nonpsychotic mental disorders
F50–F59	Behavioral syndromes associated with physiological disturbances and physical factors
F60–F69	Disorders of adult personality and behavior
F70–F79	Intellectual disabilities
F80–F89	Pervasive and specific developmental disorders
F90–F98	Behavioral and emotional disorders with onset usually occurring in childhood and adolescence
F99	Unspecified mental disorder

These conditions are generally treated by a psychologist or a psychiatrist.

The ICD-10-CM codes in this chapter are compatible with those included in the *Diagnostic and Statistical Manual of Mental Disorders, Fifth Edition Text Revision (DSM-IV-TR)*, published by the American Psychiatric Association.

Descriptions of the various diagnostic categories in *DSM-V-TR* enable clinicians and investigators to diagnose, communicate about, study, and treat people with various mental disorders. Most of the codes are the same as those used in ICD-10-CM, but the terminology may differ.

Mental Disorders Due to Known Physiological Conditions

Mental disorders (F01–F09) due to known physiological conditions are grouped together due to a demonstrable etiology in cerebral disease, brain injury, or other insults that lead to cerebral dysfunction. This cerebral dysfunction can be either primary (disease, injuries, and insults that affect the brain directly) or secondary (systemic diseases and disorders attacking the brain as one of multiple organs or systems).

There are multiple instructional notes under these categories that direct the coder to first code underlying physiological conditions or sequelae of cerebrovascular disease.

Organic Brain Syndrome

Organic brain syndrome is an old term that describes decreased mental function that is due to a medical disease rather than a psychiatric condition. Organic brain syndrome, NOS, is coded as F09, with the underlying physiological condition coded first.

Organic Anxiety Disorder

Organic anxiety disorder is considered to be the direct physiological effect of a general medical condition. Sequenced first should be the general condition along with another code, F06.4, Anxiety disorder due to known physiological condition.

Dementia

Dementia is characterized by a permanent or progressive decline in several dimensions of intellectual function that interferes with an individual's normal social or economic activity. Dementias are considered to be of physical rather than psychiatric etiology, brought about by a general medical condition, a substance, or a combination of these factors.

When dementia is present as a result of a specific underlying or physiological disease, that condition (Alzheimer's disease) is reported first, followed by a code from subcategory F02.8, Dementia in other diseases classified elsewhere.

Schizophrenic Disorders

Category F20 outlines schizophrenic disorders, referring to a group of psychoses where there is a personality disturbance or distortion of thinking, delusions, or autism.

The fourth characters refer to the type of schizophrenia—namely, paranoid, disorganized, catatonic, undifferentiated, residual, other, and unspecified—while the fifth characters further specify the fourth characters.

Affective Disorders

Affective disorders are characterized as common mental diseases with mood disturbances with multiple aspects, including biological, social, behavioral, and physiological factors.

In ICD-10-CM, affective disorders are located under categories F30–F39 and include conditions such as manic episodes, bipolar disorders, major depressive disorders, and persistent mood disorders at the fourth character level. Fifth characters further specify the above conditions.

Nonpsychotic Mental Disorders

The following types of disorders are considered nonpsychotic mental disorders:

Anxiety Disorders

Anxiety disorders are a common psychiatric problem and are one of the most undertreated problems. The fourth character levels identify manifestations of this disorder:

- F40   Phobic anxiety disorders (agoraphobia, social phobias, and specific (isolated) phobias)
- F41   Other anxiety disorders (panic disorder, generalized, and mixed anxiety disorders)
- F42   Obsessive-compulsive disorder

Fifth characters further specify some of the conditions listed in these categories.

Stress Reactions

Category F43 identifies reactions to severe stress and adjustment disorders. Code F43.0 classifies acute stress reaction and includes acute crisis reaction, acute reaction to stress, combat and operational stress reaction, combat fatigue, crisis state, and psychic shock. Posttraumatic stress disorder (PTSD) is coded to F43.1-. Fifth characters specify whether the PTSD is acute, chronic, or unspecified. Adjustment disorders such as culture shock, grief reaction, and hospitalism in children are coded to subcategory F43.2-, Adjustment disorders. Fifth characters under this code further specify the adjustment disorder such as depressed mood, anxiety, disturbances of conduct, and others.

Dissociative and Conversion Disorders

Dissociative disorders are those conditions involving disruptions or breakdown of awareness, memory, identity, or perception (for example, amnesia, fugue, stupor, and identity disorder). Category F44 classifies these conditions. Conversion disorders are those conditions when the patient presents neurological symptoms such as paralysis, speech impairment, or tremors, but with the exclusion of neurological disease or feigning, and the determination of a psychological mechanism (for example, motor symptoms or deficit, seizures or convulsions, sensory symptom or deficit, and mixed symptom presentation).

Somatoform Disorders

In ICD-10-CM, category F45 classifies somatoform disorders, which are mental disorders that are characterized by physical symptoms that tend to mimic actual physical disease or injury but without any identifiable physical cause. The diagnosis of a somatoform disorder implies that mental factors contribute to the onset, severity, and duration of any symptoms (for example, psychogenic diarrhea and dysmenorrhea, and hypochondriacal disorder).

This category also provides a code (F45.41) for pain that is exclusively related to psychological factors. The Excludes 1 note under category G89 indicates that a code from category G89 should not be assigned with code F45.41. When a patient's record documents a related psychological component for the patient's pain, two codes should be used to code this condition. Category G89, Pain, not elsewhere classified, and code F45.42.

Behavioral Syndromes Associated with Physiological Disturbances and Physical Factors

These categories (F50–F59) include behavioral syndromes associated with physiological disturbances and physical factors. These codes are not used when the conditions that present are due to a mental disorder that is of organic origin or classified elsewhere (for example, eating and sleep disorders, sexual dysfunction, or puerperal psychosis).

ICD-10-CM utilizes category F54 to classify psychological and behavioral factors that are associated with diseases that are classified elsewhere (for example, asthma, dermatitis, urticaria, and ulcerative and mucous colitis). When coding these conditions, if the condition is thought to be psychogenic in origin, the associated physical disease is the first-listed code, followed by the code F54.

Substance Abuse Disorders

In ICD-10-CM, substance abuse and dependence are considered mental disorders and are classified to categories F10–F19. The terms *abuse* and *dependence* are different conditions and thus are coded differently in ICD-10-CM.

Alcohol Abuse and Dependence

Category F10 classifies alcohol-related disorders, and there is a note to "Use additional code for blood alcohol level, if applicable (Y90.-)" immediately under this category. There is a difference between abuse and dependence. Alcohol abuse is defined as the recurring use of alcoholic beverages despite negative consequences. Alcohol dependence is a chronic condition in which a patient has become dependent on alcohol, demonstrates increased tolerance for the effects of alcohol, and is unable to stop using alcohol even when faced with strong incentives such as impaired health, deteriorating social interactions, and decreasing job performance. Such patients often experience physical signs of withdrawal during any sudden cessation of drinking. Both the terms *alcohol abuse* and *alcohol dependence* are sometimes generally referred to as alcoholism.

In ICD-10-CM, alcohol abuse is classified to subcategory F10.1, while alcohol dependence is classified to code F10.2. If alcohol use is mentioned but without the words abuse or dependence, this condition should be coded to F10.9, Alcohol use, unspecified. Fifth characters under subcategories F10.1, F10.2, and F10.9 specify the presence of intoxication, intoxication delirium, alcohol-induced mood disorder, psychotic disorder, and other alcohol-induced disorders.

Drug Dependence

Drug dependence or drug addiction is a chronic mental and physical condition related to the patient's pattern of taking a drug or a combination of drugs. Drug dependence and abuse are classified to categories F11–F19 according to the class of drug (for example, opioid, cannabis, or cocaine). Generally, fourth characters indicate whether the disorder is abuse, dependence, or unspecified, while fifth characters specify intoxication, intoxication delirium, and intoxication with perceptual disturbance. Physical complications and psychotic conditions are listed under the specific drug, with fifth and sixth characters providing information on mood disorder, psychotic disorder, withdrawal, and other drug-induced disorders.

There are also combination codes provided to indicate both alcohol and substance abuse or dependence, along with any specified complications (for example, alcoholic withdrawal delirium due to alcohol dependence, code F10.231).

Psychoactive Substance Use

ICD-10-CM provides codes for psychoactive substance use (for example, F10.9-, F11.9-) in addition to the codes for psychoactive abuse and dependence. The only time when these codes are to be used is when the psychoactive substance use is associated with a mental or behavioral disorder, and the physician must establish this relationship in the documentation.

For all substance abuse disorders, when documentation refers to *use*, *abuse*, and *dependence* of the same substance, one code should be used to identify the pattern of use and is based on the following guidelines:

- When both use and abuse are listed, assign a code for abuse.
- When both abuse and dependence are listed, use a code for the dependence.
- When both use and dependence are listed, use a code for the dependence.
- When all (use, abuse, and dependence) are listed, use a code only for dependence.

Chapter 6: ICD-10-CM Exercises

Review the following statements and cases and assign the appropriate codes:

1. Acute exacerbation of residual-type schizophrenia

2. Reactive depressive psychosis

3. Phobic anxiety reaction of childhood

4. Alcoholic gastritis due to chronic alcoholism

5. Acute senile depression

6. Attention-deficit hyperactivity disorder (ADHD)

7. Alcohol dependence syndrome in remission

8. Passive-aggressive personality disorder

9. Bipolar II disorder, NOS

10. Hypochondriac with continuous laxative habit

11. Dementia with behavioral disturbance

Continued

12. Major depression, recurrent

13. Delirium tremens (DTs) due to alcohol withdrawal

14. Schizophrenia, catatonic type

15. Alcohol abuse with intoxication

16. Unnatural fear of thunderstorms

17. Pathological pyromania

18. Asperger's syndrome

19. Borderline personality disorder, specifically described as "cluster B personality disorder." The patient is also a recovering alcoholic, which the provider describes as being "in remission."

20. A patient was brought to the ER and then admitted because of acute alcohol inebriation. Blood alcohol level shows 22 mg/100 ml. The discharge diagnosis is acute and chronic alcoholic, continuous.

Diseases of the Nervous System

After completing this lesson, you should be able to do the following:

- Apply knowledge of current ICD-10-CM coding guidelines to assign and sequence accurate codes for diagnoses related to diseases of the nervous system
- Delineate the various types of conditions related to this system
- Discuss other disorders of the brain

ICD-10-CM

Chapter 6 of the ICD-10-CM code book includes conditions that affect the brain and spinal cord as well as the peripheral nervous system.

ICD-10-CM's Chapter 6 includes the following blocks:

Categories	Section Titles
G00–G09	Inflammatory diseases of the central nervous system
G10–G14	Systemic atrophies primarily affecting the central nervous system
G20–G26	Extrapyramidal and movement disorders
G30–G32	Other degenerative diseases of the nervous system
G35–G37	Demyelinating diseases of the central nervous system
G40–G47	Episodic and paroxysmal disorders
G50–G59	Nerve, nerve root, and plexus disorders
G60–G65	Polyneuropathies and other disorders of the peripheral nervous system
G70–G73	Diseases of myoneural junction and muscle
G80–G83	Cerebral palsy and other paralytic syndromes
G89–G99	Other disorders of the nervous system

Generally, these conditions are treated by a neurologist, an ophthalmologist, or an ear, nose, and throat doctor.

Parkinson's Disease

Parkinsonism or Parkinson's disease is a progressive and chronic disorder of the central nervous system. Category G20, Parkinson's disease, includes primary parkinsonism. Category G21, Secondary parkinsonism, is often a sequela of the therapeutic use of medications; therefore, codes from T36 to T50 are assigned as first-listed codes to indicate the drug responsible, and then an appropriate code from category G21 is assigned. In some cases, syphilis causes Parkinson's disease and is coded to A52.19, Other symptomatic neurosyphilis.

Alzheimer's Disease

Alzheimer's disease is defined as a process of progressive atrophy that involves the degeneration of nerve cells and leads to changes ranging from subtle intellectual impairment to dementia. Category G30 classifies Alzheimer's disease, and this category is further divided at the fourth character level to indicate early onset, late onset, other, and unspecified. Under category G30, there is a note to "Use additional code to identify" dementia with and without behavioral disturbance. When a patient also presents with dementia, it is coded with a code from subcategory F02.8, Dementia in conditions classified elsewhere, and this is listed as an additional diagnosis.

Epilepsy

The term *epilepsy* denotes any disorder characterized by recurrent seizures. A seizure is defined as a transient disturbance of cerebral function due to an abnormal paroxysmal neuronal discharge in the brain. The terminology used to describe the different types of epilepsy has changed over the years. ICD-10-CM includes more specificity whenever possible (identifying seizures of localized onset, simple or complex, partial seizures, and intractable and status epilepticus).

Coders should be very careful using a code from category G40. This code should be assigned only when the documentation in the health record supports its use. The administration of certain anticonvulsive medication may or may not imply that a patient has epilepsy. Seizures and convulsions are not the same condition. Fifth characters under this category specify intractable and not intractable.

The physician must state "intractable epilepsy" in the health record before the fifth character can be assigned. The term *intractable* refers to the condition that is resistant to treatment. Epilepsy should never be assumed to be intractable based on generalities in the health record.

The code book includes a note under Category G40 (Epilepsy and recurrent seizures) that states that the following terms are to be considered equivalent to intractable: pharmacoresistant (pharmacologically resistant), treatment resistant, refractory (medically), and poorly controlled.

Epilepsy should never be coded unless it is stated; do not assume that if patients have seizures, they have epilepsy. Patients can experience seizures without having epilepsy. Sixth characters are used to identify whether status epilepticus is present.

Headaches and Migraines

ICD-10-CM provides codes for various types of headaches. Chapter 6, Diseases of the nervous system, includes codes for migraine (G43) and other headache syndromes (G44). Headaches without a known cause or any further specificity are included in Chapter 18, Symptoms, signs, and abnormal clinical and laboratory findings, and are coded to R51, Headache.

Many types of migraine headaches can be identified with specific codes in fourth character subcategories for migraine with aura, migraine without aura, hemiplegic migraine, persistent migraine aura with and without cerebral infarction, chronic migraine, cyclical vomiting, ophthalmoplegic migraine, periodic headache syndromes, abdominal migraine, and other forms of migraine. Category G43 requires the use of a fifth character subclassification code that specifies whether the migraine is with or without status migrainous and also whether it is intractable or not intractable. There is a note in the code book following category G43, which lists the following terms as equivalent to intractable: pharmacoresistant (pharmacologically resistant), treatment resistant, refractory (medically), and poorly controlled.

Status migrainosus is defined as headaches with a duration of greater than 72 hours. It is debilitating and incapacitating, with symptoms that typically leave the patient restricted to bed.

Hemiplegia and Hemiparesis

Hemiplegia (total paralysis) and hemiparesis (slight paralysis) are conditions characterized by paralysis of one side of the body, and it is classified to category G81. This category is further subdivided at the fourth character level to differentiate between flaccid, spastic, and unspecified hemiplegia. Flaccid refers to the loss of muscle tone in the paralyzed parts, with the absence of tendon reflexes. Spastic refers to the spasticity of the paralyzed parts, with increased tendon reflexes. These codes are often assigned when the health record provides no further information, when the cause of the hemiplegia and hemiparesis is unknown, or as an additional code when the condition results from a specified cause. The fifth character subclassification identifies the side effect and whether the affected side is dominant or nondominant. This type of specificity may not be available in the health record; if not, the coder should assign the fifth character, 0. Transient hemiplegia is a type of hemiplegia that occurs in connection with a cerebrovascular accident (CVA) and will often clear quickly. Since hemiplegia is not inherent to a CVA, a code from category G81 is used as an additional code when it does occur. If the patient is admitted some time later with hemiplegia due to sequelae of cerebrovascular disease, use a code from I69 to indicate that this condition is a sequelae of a CVA.

Pain

Encounters for pain management or for specific types of pain, such as central pain syndrome or postoperative pain, are reported with codes from category G89.

Central pain syndrome can be caused by damage to the central nervous system. This can be traumatic or brain-related (such as stroke, multiple sclerosis, tumors, epilepsy, or Parkinson's disease). This category provides a code that specifically identifies pain that is postoperative in nature. The pain can be classified as acute or chronic.

Codes in category G89 may be used in conjunction with codes from other categories and chapters to provide more detail about acute or chronic pain and neoplasm-related pain. If the pain is not specified as acute or chronic, do not assign codes from category G89 except for postthoracotomy pain, chronic postoperative pain, neoplasm-related pain, or chronic pain syndrome.

Category G89 codes are acceptable as the principal diagnosis or the first-listed code for reporting purposes when pain control or pain management is the reason for the admission or encounter. In this instance, the underlying cause of the pain should be reported as an additional diagnosis, if known.

Postoperative pain may also be reported as a secondary diagnosis code when a patient presents for outpatient surgery and subsequently develops an unusual or inordinate amount of postoperative pain. Routine or expected postoperative pain immediately after surgery should not be coded.

Codes in category G89 may also be used in conjunction with site-specific pain codes if the additional information is provided. The sequencing of these site-specific pain codes is dependent on the circumstances of the following encounters:

- If the encounter is for pain control or pain management, assign the code from category G89 followed by the code that identifies the specific pain site.

- If the encounter is for any other reason except pain control or pain management, and a related definitive diagnosis has not been established, assign the code for the specific site of the pain first, followed by the appropriate code from category G89. If the definitive diagnosis has in fact been established, then code the definitive diagnosis.

Subcategories G89.12 and G89.22 identify postthoracotomy pain, other postoperative pain, and pain due to trauma. Assignment of these codes depends on whether the pain is classified as acute or chronic.

Subcategory G89.2, Chronic pain, NEC, refers to pain that persists over a relatively long period of time. However, there is no time frame defining when pain becomes chronic pain. Refer to the physician's documentation as a guide for the use of these codes.

Code G89.3, Neoplasm-related pain, includes cancer-associated pain that may be acute or chronic, pain due to either a primary or a secondary malignancy, and tumor-associated pain. This code may be listed as the principal or first-listed code, depending on the reason for the encounter. The underlying neoplasm is reported as an additional diagnosis.

Chronic pain syndrome, code G89.4, refers to pain that persists beyond the usual recovery period with or without an identifiable cause or source. Chronic pain syndrome differs from chronic pain, so this code should be used only when the physician has specifically documented chronic pain syndrome.

Meningitis

Meningitis is the inflammation of the meninges, the three connective tissue membranes that cover the brain and spinal cord. Meningitis can be caused by a variety of microorganisms or viruses. It is classified in two chapters of the ICD-10-CM code book: Chapter 6, Diseases of the nervous system; and Chapter 1, Certain infectious and parasitic diseases. Because of this particular classification, the instructions provided in the Alphabetic Index and Tabular List must be followed to ensure accurate code assignment.

It should be noted that two codes are required in some instances, and one combination code is sufficient in others. However, accurate sequencing of the two codes is imperative. Code for the underlying condition first, and then list the manifestation code.

Brain Disorders

The brain disorders of encephalopathy, inflammatory, and toxic neuropathy are discussed below.

Inflammatory and Toxic Neuropathy

Category G60 contains different forms of polyneuritis, some of which are the result of other diseases, such as diabetes, malignancy, and collagen vascular diseases. Codes G61.1, G62.0, G62.2, and G62.82 include directions to "Use additional code for adverse effect to identify serum," "Use additional code for adverse effect to identify drug," "Use additional external cause to identify cause," and "Code first toxic agent." Fourth and fifth characters further specify each category in this section (for example, Guillain–Barre Syndrome, alcoholic polyneuropathy).

Encephalopathy

Encephalopathy describes any disorder of cerebral function and is a very broad and general term that will be preceded by other terms that describe the cause, reason, or any special conditions that may lead to a disorder of the brain. Not all terms that precede encephalopathy will be coded to Chapter 6, but a couple of common types are listed as follows:

- Alcoholic encephalopathy: complication of alcoholic liver disease and generally caused by heavy drinking for many years. It is coded to G31.2, Degeneration of nervous system due to alcohol.

- Toxic encephalopathy: also referred to as toxic-metabolic encephalopathy and is a degenerative neurologic disease caused by toxic substance exposure and is coded to category G92, Toxic encephalopathy. There is a note under this category that reminds the coder to "Code first (T51–T65) to identify toxic agent."

Chapter 7: ICD-10-CM Exercises

Review the following statements and cases and assign the appropriate codes:

1. Hemiplegia of dominant right side

2. Tonic-clonic epilepsy

3. Migraine with aura

4. *Aerobacter aerogenes* meningitis

5. Intracranial abscess

6. Generalized idiopathic epilepsy

7. Congenital diplegic cerebral palsy

8. An 88-year-old man was transferred from a local nursing home with complaints of fatigue, fever, sinus congestion, and headaches. He also suffered from Alzheimer's disease and was recently diagnosed with tic douloureux. While in the hospital, he was treated with decongestants and an antibiotic for the sinusitis.

   Discharge diagnoses: Acute frontal sinusitis; Alzheimer's disease; tic douloureux

   Code(s):

9. Treatment-resistant Lennox-Gastaut syndrome with status epilepticus

10. Entrapment of the left median nerve

11. Interdigital neuroma of right lower limb

12. Diagnosis: Secondary parkinsonism due to Haloperidol. This patient has been taking Haloperidol as prescribed for paranoid schizophrenia and developed a change in facial expressions and stiffness in the arms and legs. The drug will be discontinued.

Diseases of the Eye and Adnexa

After completing this lesson, you should be able to do the following:

- Apply knowledge of current ICD-10-CM coding guidelines to assign and sequence accurate codes for diagnoses related to diseases of the eye and adnexa
- Delineate the various conditions related to this system

ICD-10-CM

Chapter 7 of the ICD-10-CM code book includes conditions that affect the eye and adnexa. ICD-10-CM's Chapter 7 includes the following blocks:

Categories	Section Titles
H00–H05	Disorders of eyelid, lacrimal system, and orbit
H10–H11	Disorders of conjunctiva
H15–H22	Disorders of sclera, cornea, iris, and ciliary body
H25–H28	Disorders of lens
H30–H36	Disorders of choroid and retina
H40–H42	Glaucoma
H43–H44	Disorders of vitreous body and globe
H46–H47	Disorders of optic nerve and visual pathways
H49–H52	Disorders of ocular muscles, binocular movement, accommodation, and refraction
H53–H54	Visual disturbances and blindness
H55–H57	Other disorders of eye and adnexa
H59	Intraoperative and postprocedural complications and disorders of eye and adnexa, not elsewhere classified

Conjunctivitis

Category H10, Conjunctivitis, is defined as an inflammation of the conjunctiva due to allergy, infection, or some other cause. Acute conjunctivitis can also be caused by a chemical or toxic agent, and, when this is the case, assign code H10.21- along with a code from categories T51–T65 to identify the substance or chemical and then the intent (accidental and assault).

There are various conditions involving the conjunctiva:

- Vernal conjunctivitis is coded to H10.44
- Chronic giant papillary conjunctivitis (for contact lens papillary conjunctivitis) is assigned subcategory code H10.41-
- Acute toxic conjunctivitis is coded to H10.21- along with a code from categories T51–T65 (identifies chemical and intent)
- Dry eye syndrome is assigned code H04.12-

Glaucoma

Glaucoma is a group of eye diseases characterized by an increase in intraocular pressure, causing pathological changes in the optic disk and typical visual field defects. Categories H40–H42 are further subdivided to identify the various types of glaucoma. For example, patients developing glaucoma as a result of corticosteroid therapy are classified to subcategory H40.6-. Code H40.83-, Aqueous misdirection, is used to report a form of glaucoma formerly known as malignant glaucoma. When documentation in the health record states "glaucoma" only, code H40.9, Unspecified glaucoma, may be assigned. Category H40 makes use of third, fourth, and fifth characters to classify the type of glaucoma or for greater specificity. Fifth and sixth characters identify the affected eye. For some glaucoma codes (H40.20 and H40.22-), the coder should also identify the stage of the glaucoma:

0—Stage unspecified
1—Mild stage
2—Moderate stage
3—Severe stage
4—Indeterminate stage

Code Z83.511 is used to identify a family history of glaucoma and other specified eye disorders.

Cataracts

A cataract is the opacity of the crystalline lens of the eye or its capsule, resulting in a loss of vision. ICD-10-CM identifies many types of cataracts:

- Age-related cataracts
- Infantile and juvenile cataracts
- Traumatic cataracts
- Complicated cataracts
- Drug-induced cataracts
- Secondary cataracts

Code assignment is not based on the age of the patient but rather the documentation of the diagnosis by the care provider. When coding cataracts, the coder should be aware of the terminology used in the diagnosis. Cataracts in patients with diabetes are usually senile or age-related. When documentation in the health record states "cataract" only, code H26.9, Unspecified cataract, should be assigned.

Chapter 8: ICD-10-CM Exercises

Review the following statements and cases and assign the appropriate codes:

1. Partial left retinal detachment with single retinal defect

2. Acute follicular conjunctivitis, right eye

3. Senile or age-related cataract

4. A 78-year-old man was seen in the physician's office for his annual eye examination. During the examination, it was discovered that he had a mature, asymptomatic senile cataract in his right eye. Moreover, the intraocular pressure in that eye was not within normal limits. The physician's recommendation was to have the patient schedule surgery for removal of the cataract.

   Impression: Mature cataract, right eye, primary open-angle glaucoma with borderline findings, low tension

   Code(s):

5. An eighth grade student was seen in the physician's office, because she was no longer able to clearly see the blackboard from her seat near the back of the classroom. After her eyes were dilated and examined, the physician determined that she was nearsighted and prescribed glasses to correct the problem.

   Impression: Myopia

   Code(s):

6. Neurogenic ptosis of right eyelid

7. Convergent concomitant strabismus, left eye

8. The patient visited her ophthalmologist and reports that she thinks she has a problem, since she has begun to see black spots in the visual field of her right eye. The physician examines the patient and diagnoses a retinal detachment with no break.

9. A mother brings her daughter to the physician's office because the child's eyes are red, itching, and swollen. The physician examines the child and diagnoses pinkeye.

10. The patient presents complaining of what looks like a stye near the corner of her right eye on the lower lid. The doctor confirms her suspicion and diagnoses a stye.

11. Primary open-angle glaucoma of the left eye

12. Ectropion due to a cicatrix on the right lower eyelid

Diseases of the Ear and Mastoid Process

OBJECTIVES

After completing this lesson, you should be able to do the following:

- Apply knowledge of current ICD-10-CM coding guidelines to assign and sequence accurate codes for diagnoses related to diseases of the ear and mastoid process
- Delineate the various conditions related to this system

ICD-10-CM

Chapter 8 of the ICD-10-CM code book includes conditions that affect the ear and mastoid process. ICD-10-CM's Chapter 8 includes the following blocks:

Categories	Section Titles
H60–H62	Diseases of external ear
H65–H75	Diseases of middle ear and mastoid
H80–H83	Diseases of inner ear
H90–H94	Other disorders of ear
H95	Intraoperative and postprocedural complications and disorders of ear and mastoid process, not elsewhere classified

Otitis

The following types of otitis are discussed as follows:

Otitis Externa

Otitis externa (external otitis), including swimmer's ear, is an infection of the external auditory canal and may be acute or chronic. Acute otitis externa is characterized by moderate to severe pain, fever, regional cellulitis, and partial hearing loss. Instead of pain, chronic otitis externa is characterized by pruritus, which leads to scaling and thickening of the skin.

ICD-10-CM classifies otitis externa to categories H60, Otitis externa, and H60.8-, Other otitis externa. Both H60 and H60.8 are further subdivided with fifth and sixth characters, which offer more specificity.

Otitis Media

Otitis media (OM) is an inflammation of the middle ear that may be further specified as suppurative or secretory and acute or chronic. Acute suppurative OM is characterized by severe, deep, throbbing pain; sneezing and coughing; mild to high fever; hearing loss, dizziness, and nausea and vomiting. Acute secretory OM results in severe conductive hearing loss and, in some cases, a sensation of fullness in the ear with popping, crackling, or clicking sounds on swallowing or with jaw movement. Chronic OM has its origin in the childhood years but usually persists into adulthood. Cumulative effects of chronic OM include thickening and scarring of the tympanic membrane, decreased or absent tympanic mobility, cholesteatoma, and painless purulent discharge.

ICD-10-CM classifies OM to categories H65 and H66. Both categories are further subdivided to identify acute, subacute, chronic forms, and other specific types of OM.

Hearing Loss and Deafness

Hearing loss may be bilateral or unilateral and is classified as follows:

- Subcategories H90.0–H90.2—Conductive or Conductive Deafness—caused by a defect in the conductive apparatus of the ear
- Subcategory H90.3–H90.5—Sensorineural—caused by a defect in the sensory mechanism of the ear/nerves
- Subcategories H90.6–H90.8—Mixed conductive and sensorineural hearing loss (combination of above two types)

Hearing loss may also be classified according to the underlying cause, such as ingestion of toxic substances, presbycusis, and sudden idiopathic hearing loss.

Chapter 9: ICD-10-CM Exercises

Review the following statements and cases and assign the appropriate codes:

1. Chronic serous otitis media

2. Cholesteatoma of middle ear

3. Congenital external microtia

4. Sensory hearing loss

5. Perforation of tympanic membrane

6. Patulous eustachian tube, left ear

7. A child is brought to the physician's office because his left ear is hurting. He has been taking swimming lessons, and the mother fears he may have an infection. The ENT doctor takes a look and diagnoses his condition as Swimmer's ear, and he prescribes drops for the child to use.

8. A patient is seen by the doctor for complaints of pain in both ears. He states that he has had some difficulty hearing lately and the sounds he does hear are muffled. The physician checks both ears and discovers impacted ear wax and removes the wax from both ears. Code only the diagnosis, not the removal of the wax.

9. A mother brings her child to the walk-in clinic because the baby has been crying and pulling on her left ear. She recently had an ear infection in the same ear, so the mother suspects this may be the case again. The doctor examines the child's ear and diagnoses recurrent acute suppurative otitis media without spontaneous rupture of eardrum.

10. Bilateral conductive hearing loss in both ears due to nonobliterative otosclerosis of the stapes at the oval window. She is unable to hear with hearing aids and has decided to undergo left stapedectomy. During the surgery, an inadvertent laceration was made to the tympanic meatal flap, which was repaired. Assign the diagnosis codes only.

Diseases of the Circulatory System

Chapter

10

OBJECTIVES

After completing this lesson, you should be able to do the following:

- Apply knowledge of current ICD-10-CM coding guidelines to assign and sequence accurate codes related to diseases of the circulatory system
- Delineate the major types of circulatory disorders
- Differentiate between the different conditions regarded as ischemic heart disease
- Understand the difference between systolic and diastolic heart failure

ICD-10-CM

Chapter 9 of the ICD-10-CM code book provides a separate group of diagnostic codes for disorders of the circulatory system. These disorders are generally treated by cardiologists and cardiovascular surgeons.

ICD-10-CM Chapter 9, Diseases of the circulatory system (I00–I99) includes the following blocks:

Categories	Section Titles
I00–I02	Acute rheumatic fever
I05–I09	Chronic rheumatic heart diseases
I10–I15	Hypertensive diseases
I20–I25	Ischemic heart diseases
I26–I28	Pulmonary heart disease and diseases of pulmonary circulation
I30–I52	Other forms of heart disease
I60–I69	Cerebrovascular diseases
I70–I79	Diseases of arteries, arterioles, and capillaries
I80–I89	Diseases of veins, lymphatic vessels, and lymph nodes, not elsewhere classified
I95–I99	Other and unspecified disorders of the circulatory system

Circulatory system codes are often difficult to apply because a variety of nonspecific terminology is used to describe circulatory conditions. The coder should carefully review all the inclusion and exclusion notes in this chapter before assigning a code.

Valvular Heart Disease

Valvular heart disease occurs in different forms. Three types of mechanical disruption can occur: stenosis, or narrowing of the valve opening; incomplete closure of the valve; or prolapse of the valve. These conditions can result from disorders such as endocarditis, congenital defects, and inflammation, and may be coded as rheumatic or nonrheumatic. ICD-10-CM provides codes that specify single- or multiple-valve involvement.

Acute Rheumatic Fever and Rheumatic Heart Disease

Acute and chronic diseases of rheumatic origin are classified to categories I00–I02. This section also covers diseases of mitral and aortic valves.

Acute Rheumatic Fever

Rheumatic fever occurs after a streptococcal sore throat (group A *Streptococcus hemolyticus*). The acute phase of the illness is marked by fever, malaise, sweating, palpitations, and polyarthritis, which varies from vague discomfort to severe pain felt chiefly in the large joints. Most patients have elevated titers of antistreptolysin antibodies and increased erythrocyte sedimentation rates.

The importance of rheumatic fever derives entirely from its capacity to cause severe heart damage. Salicylates markedly reduce fever, relieve joint pain, and may reduce joint swelling when present. Because rheumatic fever often recurs, prophylaxis with penicillin is recommended and has markedly reduced the incidence of rheumatic heart disease in the general population.

Chronic Rheumatic Heart Disease

Rheumatic heart disease develops with an initial attack of rheumatic fever in about 30 percent of cases. The cardiac involvement may affect all three layers, causing pericarditis, scarring and weakening of the myocardium, and endocardial involvement of heart valves. A murmur heard over the heart is symptomatic of a valvular lesion. Rheumatic fever causes inflammation of the valves, thus damaging the valve cusps, so that the opening may become permanently narrowed (stenosis). The mitral valve is involved in 75 to 80 percent of such cases; the aortic valve in 30 percent; and the tricuspid and pulmonary valves in less than 5 percent. In about 10 percent of patients, two of these valves are involved.

When stenosis affects the mitral valve, blood flow decreases from the left atrium into the left ventricle. As a result, blood is held back, first in the lungs, then in the right side of the heart, and, finally, in the veins of the body. Incompetence of a valve also may occur because the cusps will not retract. When the mitral valve cannot close, blood escapes back into the left atrium from the mitral valve. When the aortic valve cannot close, blood escapes from the aorta into the left ventricle. In such cases, plastic and metal replacement valves that function as well as normal valves may be inserted surgically.

In coding diseases of the mitral valve and diseases affecting both the mitral and aortic valves, the Alphabetic Index offers direction to specific codes. Remember to always trust the Alphabetic Index and assign the code it indicates. Generally ICD-10-CM does presume that a disorder affecting both the aortic and mitral valves is rheumatic in origin. Otherwise, the aortic condition is presumed to be rheumatic only when the diagnosis specifically states "rheumatic." Certain mitral valve disorders (when the etiology is unknown) are presumed to be rheumatic in origin. When more than one condition affects the mitral valve and one is stated to be rheumatic, then all are classified as rheumatic.

When a patient with a diagnosis of heart failure also has rheumatic heart disease, it is classified as rheumatic heart failure (I09.81), unless, of course, the physician directs otherwise. There is a note under code I09.81 that directs the coder to "Use additional code to identify type of heart failure."

Hypertension

Benign Hypertension

In most cases, benign hypertension remains fairly stable over many years and is compatible with a long life. When untreated, however, it becomes an important risk factor in coronary artery disease and cerebrovascular disease. Benign hypertension is also asymptomatic, until complications develop. Effective antihypertensive drug therapy is the treatment of choice.

Malignant Hypertension

Malignant hypertension (also known as accelerated hypertension) is far less common, occurring in only about 1 percent of patients with elevated blood pressure. The malignant form is frequently of abrupt onset and runs a course measured in months. It often ends with renal failure or cerebral hemorrhage. Usually a person with malignant hypertension will complain of headaches and difficulties with vision. Blood pressure is extremely high in malignant hypertension, and an abnormal protrusion of the optic nerve (papilledema) occurs with microscopic hemorrhages and exudates seen in the retina. The chances for long-term survival depend on prompt treatment before organ damage occurs.

Hypertensive Heart Disease

Hypertensive heart disease refers to the secondary effects on the heart of prolonged, sustained, systemic hypertension. The heart has to work against greatly increased resistance in the form of high blood pressure. The primary effect is thickening of the left ventricle, finally resulting in heart failure. The symptoms are similar to those of heart failure from other causes. Many persons with controlled hypertension do not develop heart failure. However, when a patient has heart failure due to hypertension, follow the instructional note with category I11 regarding use of an additional code to specify the type of heart failure that exists, if known.

Chapter-Specific Coding Guidelines

The following guidelines are applicable in coding hypertensive diseases:

- **Hypertension, essential:** Assign hypertension (essential) (systemic) to category I10.
- **Hypertension with heart disease:** Heart conditions (I50.- or I51.4–I51.9) are assigned to a code from category I11 when a causal relationship is stated or implied. Use an additional code from to identify the type of heart failure in those patients with heart failure.

  The same conditions (I50.-, I51.4–I51.9) with hypertension but without a stated causal relationship between the hypertension and heart condition are coded separately. The coder should sequence the codes according to the circumstances of the admission or encounter.

  In ICD-10-CM, a stated causal relationship is usually documented using the term *due to* (for example, congestive heart failure due to hypertension). An implied causal relationship is documented using the term *hypertensive*. In ICD-10-CM, hypertensive is interpreted to mean *due to*. Therefore, hypertensive cardiomegaly also can be described as cardiomegaly due to hypertension.
- **Hypertensive chronic kidney disease (CKD):** Assign codes from category I12, Hypertensive chronic kidney disease, when conditions classified to category N18 (CKD) and

hypertension are present. Unlike hypertension with heart disease, ICD-10-CM presumes a cause-and-effect relationship and classifies CKD with hypertension as hypertensive CKD. A code from category N18 should be used to as a secondary code along with a code from category I12 in order to identify the stage of CKD.

- **Hypertensive heart and CKD:** Assign codes from category I13, Hypertensive heart and chronic kidney disease, when both hypertensive kidney disease and hypertensive heart disease are specifically stated in the final diagnosis. One can assume a causal relationship between the hypertension and the CKD, whether the condition is designated that way. If there is a presence of heart failure, an additional code from category I50 should be assigned in order to identify the type of heart failure. A code from category N18 would be used as a secondary code along with category code I13 in order to specify the stage of CKD.

  Pay particular attention to the Includes note under category I13, as it states that it includes any condition in I11 with any condition in I12. If a patient has CKD and acute renal failure, then an additional code for the acute renal failure is needed.

- **Hypertensive cerebrovascular disease:** Two codes are required to fully describe a hypertensive cerebrovascular condition. The first code assigned describes the cerebrovascular disease (I60–I69), followed by the appropriate code describing the hypertension.

- **Hypertensive retinopathy:** Two codes are required to identify hypertensive retinopathy. First, assign code H35.0, Background retinopathy and retinal vascular change, followed by the appropriate code from categories I10 describing the hypertension.

- **Hypertension, secondary:** When a physician documents that the hypertension is due to another disease (secondary hypertension), two codes are required to describe the condition completely. One code describes the underlying condition, and the other is selected from category I15, Secondary hypertension. Sequencing of codes is determined by the reason for encounter or admission.

- **Hypertension, transient, and elevated blood pressure:** Assign code R03.0, Elevated blood pressure reading without diagnosis of hypertension, when the diagnosis states either "elevated blood pressure reading" or "transient elevated blood pressure reading." When the patient has a diagnosis of hypertension, also assign a code for the hypertension.

- **Controlled hypertension:** Assign the appropriate code from categories I10–I15 to describe a diagnostic statement of controlled hypertension. This type of statement usually refers to an existing state of hypertension under control by therapy.

Ischemic Heart Disease

Ischemic heart disease (categories I20–I25) includes arteriosclerotic heart disease, coronary ischemia, and coronary artery disease. It is the generic name for three forms of heart disease: myocardial infarction (MI), angina pectoris, and chronic ischemic heart disease. All three diseases result from an imbalance between the need of the myocardium for oxygen and the oxygen supply. Usually the imbalance results from insufficient blood flow due to arteriosclerotic narrowing of the coronary arteries.

Myocardial Infarction

MI usually occurs as a result of sudden inadequacy of coronary blood flow. One common symptom of acute MI is the development of deep substernal pain described as an ache or pressure, often with radiation to the back or left arm. The patient is pale, diaphoretic (sweaty), and in severe pain. Major complications include tachycardia, frequent ventricular premature beats, Mobitz II heart block, and ventricular fibrillation. Heart failure occurs in about two-thirds of hospitalized MI patients. MI is reported with a code from category I21, ST elevation myocardial infarction (STEMI) and non-ST elevation myocardial infarction (NSTEMI). The fourth character describes the specific location affected in the heart (that is, lateral wall or anterior wall).

An MI is described as acute if it has a duration of four weeks or less. Subcategory codes I21.0–I21.2 have a fifth character that describes which coronary artery is involved. Transmural infarctions are identified by codes I21.0- through I21.3-. If an acute myocardial infarction (AMI) is documented as transmural or subendocardial, but the site is provided, it is still coded as a subendocardial AMI.

If a patient requires continued care for a MI after the four-week time frame, then an appropriate aftercare code would be used instead of a code from category I21. For an old or healed MI that does not require further care, assign code I25.2, Old MI.

If a patient suffers a new MI with four weeks of an acute MI, use a code from category I22, STEMI and NSTEMI, in conjunction with a code from category I21.

Diagnostic Tools

The diagnosis of AMI depends on the patient's clinical history, the physical examination, interpretation of electrocardiogram (EKG), chest radiograph, and measurement of serum levels of cardiac enzymes.

Diagnostic uncertainty frequently arises because of various factors. Many patients with AMI have atypical symptoms. Other patients with typical physical symptoms do not have AMI. EKGs may also be nondiagnostic. Laboratory tests known as biochemical or serum markers of cardiac injury are commonly relied upon to diagnose or exclude an AMI.

Creatine kinase and lactate dehydrogenase have been the gold standard for the diagnosis of AMI for many years. However, single values of these tests have limited sensitivity and specificity. Newer serum markers currently in use are troponin T and I, myoglobin, and the MB isoenzyme of creatine kinase. These markers are now being used instead of, or along with, the standard markers.

EKGs also prove useful in the diagnosis of MIs. The initial EKG may be diagnostic in acute transmural MI, but serial EKGs may be necessary to confirm the diagnosis for other MI sites.

A patient diagnosed with an acute MI or an acute ischemic stroke may be given intravenous tissue plasminogen activator (tPA), which is a thrombolytic agent also known as a clot-busting drug. Studies have shown that tPA and other clot-dissolving agents can reduce the amount of damage to the heart muscle and save lives. In order to be effective, tPA must be given within the first three hours after the onset of symptoms.

Evolving Infarction

A MI described as evolving will sometimes precipitate right ventricular failure that then progresses to congestive heart failure. The first-listed diagnosis in this case would be the infarction, with an additional code for the heart failure. If cardiogenic shock, ventricular arrhythmia, and fibrillation are mentioned, these conditions should also be coded.

Other Acute and Subacute Ischemic Heart Diseases

Angina

Angina may be classified as either unstable angina or angina pectoris. Unstable angina may also be described as crescendo, accelerated, denovo effort, intermediate coronary syndrome, worsening effort, or preinfarction angina and is the development of prolonged episodes of anginal discomfort, usually occurring at rest and requiring hospitalization to rule out MI. Unstable angina is classified to code I20.0.

When there is a diagnosis of acute ischemic heart disease or acute myocardial ischemia, it does not always indicate an infarction. When there is occlusion or thrombosis of the artery without infarction, code either I24.0 or I24.8.

Chronic Ischemic Heart Disease

Arteriosclerosis or atherosclerosis is the narrowing of an arterial wall caused by the deposition of plaque-forming cholesterol and other lipids within the lumen. The large arteries—the aorta and its main branches—are primarily affected, but smaller arteries, such as the coronary and cerebral arteries, also can be affected. The patient experiences chest pain, shortness of breath, and sweating. Blood pressure is high; pulse is rapid and weak. An x-ray reveals cardiomegaly and narrowing, or occlusion, of the affected vessel wall. Blood tests may show hypercholesterolemia.

Atherosclerosis is the major cause of ischemia of the heart, brain, and extremities. Its complications include stroke, congestive heart failure, angina pectoris, MI, and kidney failure. Coronary atherosclerosis is reported with subcategory I25.1-, which is further expanded to identify involvement of the native coronary arteries and bypassed grafts. The fifth character codes are vessel-specific and should be assigned when the physician's documentation states that atherosclerosis has been found in that specific vessel.

- Code I25.9 is assigned when the documentation in the health record does not indicate whether the disease is present in a native vessel or a graft in a patient who has previously undergone aortocoronary bypass surgery or in a patient whose surgical history is unknown.

- Code I25.1- is assigned to show coronary artery disease in a native coronary artery.

- Code I25.71- is assigned to show coronary artery disease in an autologous vein bypass graft with angina pectoris.

- Code I25.72- is assigned when the physician documents the diagnosis of coronary atherosclerosis in an internal mammary artery or other artery used for a bypass graft.

- Code I25.73- is assigned to show coronary artery disease in a nonautologous biological bypass graft.

- Code I25.810 is assigned when the physician documents the diagnosis of coronary atherosclerosis in a bypass graft without angina pectoris. This code is used when there is no further documentation of the type of bypass graft used.

- Code I25.811 is assigned when there is evidence of coronary atherosclerosis in the native coronary arteries of a patient who has had a heart transplant.

- Code I25.812 is assigned when there is evidence of coronary atherosclerosis in the bypass graft of a patient who has had a heart transplant without angina pectoris.

- Code I25.82 is used to indicate chronic total occlusion of a coronary artery. The coder is instructed to "Code first coronary atherosclerosis."

- Code I25.83 is used to indicate coronary atherosclerosis due to lipid rich plaque. The coder is also instructed to "Code first coronary atherosclerosis."

Subcategory code I25.89 refers to other specified forms of chronic ischemic heart disease.

Heart Failure

Heart failure is characterized by the inability of the heart to contract with enough force to pump blood properly. It may be caused by hypertension, incompetent heart valves, or weakness of the heart resulting from MI. Heart failure may develop gradually or occur acutely. Its effects include the following:

- Increased pressure in the lung as fluid collects in the lung tissue, inhibiting oxygen and carbon dioxide exchange
- Impaired kidney function as blood filters poorly and body sodium and water retention increase, resulting in edema
- Impaired blood circulation as fluid collects in tissues, resulting in edema of the feet and legs

Early signs of heart failure are tachycardia, fatigue, dyspnea with exertion, nocturnal dyspnea, cough, and intolerance to cold. Symptoms deteriorate into a productive, blood-tinged cough, wheezing, feelings of suffocation, and cyanosis. Patients are pale and perspiring, with moist rales heard at the base of the lungs. Respiration becomes labored and weak, with a rapid pulse and congested lungs with oliguria. ICD-10-CM classifies two main categories of heart failure: systolic heart failure (I50.2-) and diastolic heart failure (I50.3-). Fifth characters specify whether the heart failure is unspecified, acute, chronic, or acute on chronic. Heart failure is further differentiated clinically by whether the right or left ventricle is affected (code I50.1), Left ventricular failure or Right-sided failure, code I50.9, Heart failure, unspecified.

Diagnostic Tests

Several diagnostic tests are important in diagnosing heart failure. Typical remarks on a chest x-ray include hilar congestion, butterfly or batwing appearance of vascular markings, bronchial edema, Kerley B lines signifying chronic elevation of left atrial pressure, and heart enlargement. An echocardiograph measures the amount of blood pumped from the heart with each beat. This measurement is known as the ejection fraction. A normal heart pumps one half (50 percent) or more of the blood in the left ventricle with each heartbeat. With heart failure, the weakened heart may pump 40 percent or less, and less blood is pumped with less force to all parts of the body.

Vital capacity (amount of air that can be expelled from the lungs) is reduced. Oxygen content of the blood is reduced, and circulation time is longer (normal circulation time from arm to lung is four to eight seconds).

Urinalysis results show slight albuminuria, increased concentration with specific gravity of 1.020, and urine sodium decreased. Laboratory findings may include blood urea nitrogen (BUN) 60 mg/100 ml; acidosis pH <7.35 due to increased CO_2 in blood from pulmonary insufficiency; and increased blood volume with a decrease in chloride, albumin, and total protein.

Cardiomyopathy

Cardiomyopathy is a disease, often of an unknown cause, that involves the muscle of the heart. ICD-10-CM classifies most cardiomyopathies to category I42.-, with the fourth characters identifying specific types:

- I42.0 Dilated cardiomyopathy
- I42.1 Obstructive hypertrophic cardiomyopathy
- I42.2 Other hypertrophic cardiomyopathy
- I42.3 Endomyocardial (eosinophilic) disease
- I42.4 Endocardial fibroelastosis
- I42.5 Other restrictive cardiomyopathy
- I42.6 Alcoholic cardiomyopathy

- I42.7   Cardiomyopathy due to drug and external agent
- I42.8   Other cardiomyopathies
- I42.9   Cardiomyopthy, unspecified

The underlying cause, such as a nutritional disorder, should be reported first if the cardiomyopathy is due to an underlying cause. Ischemic cardiomyopathy, resulting from prolonged, persistent deficiency of blood to the heart muscle, is reported with code I25.5, Ischemic cardiomyopathy.

Cardiac Dysrhythmias

Cardiac dysrhythmias identify disturbances or impairments of the normal electrical activity of heart muscle excitation. ICD-10-CM classifies cardiac dysrhythmias to several categories, depending on the specific type. Without further specification as to type of cardiac dysrhythmia, code I49.9 may be reported. Some common dysrhythmias are discussed here:

- Atrial fibrillation (I48.91) is commonly associated with organic heart disease, such as coronary artery disease, hypertension and rheumatic mitral valve disease, thyrotoxicosis, pericarditis, and pulmonary embolism. Treatment includes pharmacologic therapy (verapamil, digoxin, and propranolol) and cardioversion.

- Atrial flutter (I48.92) is associated with ischemic heart disease and pulmonary disease. Treatment is similar to the treatment for atrial fibrillation.

- Ventricular fibrillation (I49.01) involves no cardiac output and is associated with cardiac arrest. Treatment is consistent with the treatment for cardiac arrest.

- Paroxysmal supraventricular tachycardia (I47.-) is associated with congenital accessory atrial conduction pathway, physical or psychological stress, hypoxia, hypokalemia, caffeine and marijuana use, stimulant use, and digitalis toxicity. Treatment includes pharmacologic therapy (quinidine, propranolol, and verapamil) and cardioversion.

- Sick sinus syndrome (I49.5), often abbreviated as SSS, has various characteristics and an imprecise diagnosis. It may be diagnosed when the patient presents with sinus arrest, sinoatrial exit block, or persistent sinus bradycardia. Often SSS is the result of drug therapy, including digitalis, calcium channel blockers, beta blockers, sympatholytic agents, and antiarrhythmic agents. Another presentation includes recurrent supraventricular tachycardia associated with bradyarrhythmias. Prolonged ambulatory monitoring may be indicated to establish a diagnosis of SSS. Treatment includes insertion of a permanent cardiac pacemaker.

- Wolff-Parkinson-White syndrome (I45.6), often abbreviated as WPW, is caused by conduction from the sinoatrial node to the ventricle through an accessory pathway that bypasses the atrioventricular (AV) node. Patients with WPW syndrome present with tachyarrhythmias, including supraventricular tachycardia and atrial fibrillation or flutter. Treatment includes catheter ablation following electrophysiologic evaluation.

- AV heart blocks are classified as being of first, second, or third degree:
  - First-degree AV block is associated with atrial septal defects or valvular disease. ICD-10-CM classifies first-degree AV block to code I44.0.
  - Second-degree AV block is further classified as follows: Mobitz type I (Wenckebach) is associated with acute inferior wall MI or digitalis toxicity. Treatment includes discontinuation of digitalis and administration of atropine. ICD-10-CM classifies Mobitz type I AV block to code I44.1. Mobitz type II is associated with anterior wall or anteroseptal MI and digitalis toxicity. Treatment includes temporary pacing and, in some cases, permanent pacemaker insertion, as well as discontinuation of digitalis and administration of atropine. ICD-10-CM classifies Mobitz type II AV block to code I44.1.

- Third-degree AV block, also referred to as complete heart block, is associated with ischemic heart disease or infarction, postsurgical complication of mitral valve replacement, digitalis toxicity, and Stokes-Adams syndrome. Treatment includes permanent cardiac pacemaker insertion. ICD-10-CM classifies third-degree AV block to code I44.2. When this type of heart block is congenital in nature, code Q24.6 is reported rather than I44.2.
- Sinus tachycardia is associated with normal physiologic response to fever, exercise, anxiety, pain, and dehydration. It also may accompany shock, left ventricular failure, cardiac tamponade, anemia, hyperthyroidism, hypovolemia, pulmonary embolism, and anterior MI. Treatment is geared toward correcting the underlying cause. ICD-10-CM classifies paroxysmal sinus tachycardia, as well as supraventricular tachycardia, to code I47.1.

Cardiac Arrest

Cardiac arrest, code I46.9 (excluding cardiac arrest that occurs with pregnancy, anesthesia overdose or wrong substance given, and postoperative complications), may be assigned as a principal diagnosis under the following circumstance:

- The patient arrives in the hospital in a state of cardiac arrest and cannot be resuscitated, or is only briefly resuscitated, and is pronounced dead, with the underlying cause of the cardiac arrest not established or unknown. This applies whether the patient is seen only in the emergency department or is admitted to the hospital, and the underlying cause is not determined prior to death.

Cardiac arrest may be used as a secondary diagnosis in the following situations:

- The patient arrives at the hospital's emergency department in a state of cardiac arrest and is resuscitated and admitted with the condition prompting the cardiac arrest known, such as trauma or ventricular tachycardia. The condition causing the cardiac arrest is sequenced first, with the cardiac arrest code listed as a secondary code. Note that codes are not assigned for symptoms integral to the condition.
- When cardiac arrest occurs during the course of the hospital stay, and the patient is resuscitated, code I46.9 may be used as a secondary code.
- When the physician documents cardiac arrest to describe an inpatient death, code I46.9 should not be assigned when the underlying cause or contributing cause of death is known.

Cardiac arrest can also occur as a complication of surgery. In that case, it is coded as I97.710, Intraoperative cardiac arrest during cardiac surgery.

Cerebrovascular Disease

Cerebrovascular disease (categories I60–I69) is any condition affecting the cerebral arteries, including hemorrhage, occlusion, and thrombosis. ICD-10-CM classifies cerebrovascular disease according to type of condition, as follows:

- I60   Nontraumatic subarachnoid hemorrhage
- I61   Nontraumatic intracerebral hemorrhage
- I62   Other and unspecified nontraumatic intracranial hemorrhage
- I63   Cerebral infarction
- I65   Occlusion and stenosis of precerebral arteries, not resulting in cerebral infarction
- I66   Occlusion and stenosis of cerebral arteries, not resulting in cerebral infarction
- I67   Other cerebrovascular diseases

- I68   Cerebrovascular disorders in diseases classified elsewhere
- I69   Sequelae of cerebrovascular disease

Subcategory I63.9, Cerebral infarction, unspecified, is assigned when the diagnosis states cerebrovascular accident (CVA) without further specification. The health record should be reviewed carefully to ensure that nothing more specific is available. Postoperative CVA is reported using codes I97.820, Postprocedural cerebrovascular infarction during cardiac surgery, or I97.821, Postprocedural cerebrovascular infarction during other surgery.

Category I69, Sequelae of cerebrovascular disease, is further subdivided to identify the specific effect; for example, hemiplegia or monoplegia, aphasia, dysphagia, or facial weakness.

Fourth-character subclassifications indicate a causal condition (nontraumatic subarachnoid hemorrhage and intracerebral hemorhage). Fifth characters provide information about the neurological deficits, such as unspecified sequelae, cognitive deficits, speech and language deficits, monoplegia of upper and lower limbs, hemiplegia/hemiparesis, other paralytic syndrome, and other sequelae.

When the documentation in the health record indicates sequelae of cerebrovascular diseases without further specification about type, code I69.9-, Sequelae of unspecified cerebrovascular disease, may be reported.

When the health record documentation indicates an old CVA with no neurologic deficits, assign code Z86.73. In this chapter, take care to carefully review all notes for instructions to "Use additional codes."

Diseases of Arteries, Arterioles, and Capillaries

The Diseases of the Arteries, Arterioles, and Capillaries section includes categories I70–I79. Some of the conditions belonging to this section are described here.

Atherosclerosis of the Peripheral Extremities

Atherosclerosis of the peripheral extremities is classified to category I70, which is further subdivided to describe the progression of the disease with intermittent claudication (I70.21), rest pain (I70.22), ulceration (I70.23), or gangrene (I70.26). Notations appearing below codes I70.23–I70.26 remind the coder that as the disease progresses, the code describing the severity of any ulcer is reported. Code I70.92 should be used as an additional code with subcategories I70.2–I70.7 when a chronic total occlusion is present with arteriosclerosis of the extremities.

Peripheral Vascular Disease

ICD-10-CM classifies other specified peripheral vascular diseases (PVDs) to category I73.8-, which is further subdivided to identify specific types for example, erythromelalgia. Without further specification, PVD is reported with code I73.9.

Arterial Embolism and Thrombosis of Extremities

Arterial embolism and thrombosis of extremities are reported with category code I74, with the fourth characters specifying the specific site and the fifth characters further specifying fourth character codes. An embolism is a blood clot or foreign substance blocking an artery that was brought to its site of blockage by blood current. A thrombosis is an abnormal aggregation of blood factors causing an arterial obstruction. A thrombus is a stationary blood clot as opposed to the embolus, which travels to its site of blockage. Atheroembolism, obstruction of a blood vessel by a cholesterol-containing embolism, is reported with category I75, Atheroembolism. Saddle emboli are one of the most severe type of emboli. The most common site for a saddle embolus is the aorta (code I75.01-), but they can occur at other sites. Coders should also review codes I75.0- through I75.89.

Pulmonary Embolism

Category I26 classifies an acute pulmonary embolism. It contains fourth characters, which indicate whether there is acute cor pulmonale, while fifth characters indicate septic and saddle pulmonary emboli. An embolus is defined as a blood clot occurring most often in veins of the leg(s), which is referred to as deep vein thrombosis (DVT). An embolus can dislodge and is then carried to other parts of the body. Anticoagulants (heparin, Coumadin) are the method of treatment for acute emboli.

Clots can also lodge in the lungs causing a condition known as pulmonary embolism. These emboli can be either acute or chronic and are coded as follows:

- I26, Pulmonary embolism, for acute pulmonary emboli: fourth characters indicate whether there is acute cor pulmonale, while fifth characters are indicative of septic pulmonary embolism.
- I27.82, Chronic pulmonary embolism, for chronic or recurring pulmonary embolism. A code for long-term (current) use of anticoagulants (Z79.01) must also be assigned for the associated long-term use of this drug.

Chapter 10: ICD-10-CM Exercises

Review the following statements and cases and assign the appropriate codes:

1. Mitral valve stenosis with aortic valve insufficiency

2. Hypertensive stage IV CKD

3. Old MI

4. This same patient (from exercise #3) presented to the emergency department two weeks later and was diagnosed with an acute inferior wall MI. She is still being monitored following her initial heart attack three weeks earlier and continues to have atrial fibrillation.

5. Acute subendocardial infarction, initial episode

6. Acute systolic heart failure; benign essential hypertension

7. Hypertension due to Cushing's disease

8. Congestive heart failure and end-stage renal disease due to accelerated hypertension

9. Acute CVA due to stenosis and infarction of right carotid artery

10. Arteriosclerosis of right lower leg with intermittent claudication

11. AV block, Mobitz type II

Continued

12. Hypertensive cardiomegaly

13. Acute coronary insufficiency

14. A patient presents for treatment and is diagnosed with aortic stenosis and mitral valve regurgitation.

15. The patient comes to the cardiologist's office and comments that her hypertension does not seem to be responding to her current medication. Her blood pressure is normal at one reading and an hour later can be extremely high. This fluctuation goes on throughout the day. The physician diagnoses this patient as having uncontrolled hypertension.

16. Acute non-ST anterior wall MI. Atrial fibrillation.

17. Thrombophlebitis of right femoral vein

18. Varicose veins of lower extremities with inflammation

19. Mesenteric lymphadenitis

20. Six months ago the patient was diagnosed with a thoracoabdominal aortic aneurysm and returns to the physician's office today to have this condition checked out. The necessary testing was done, and the physician concludes that the aneurysm is still rather small and tells the patient that he will check it again in a few months. His diagnosis is thoracoabdominal aortic aneurysm.

21. A patient is diagnosed with cardiac tamponade due to viral pericarditis.

22. A patient is seen with arteriosclerotic heart disease.

23. Progressive episodes of chest pain determined to be crescendo angina. The patient has no previous history of CABG. He had MI five years ago and was diagnosed with coronary artery disease and progressively has been having more frequent episodes of chest pain.

24. Pulmonary hypertension due to cor pulmonale

Chapter

11

Diseases of the Respiratory System

OBJECTIVES

After completing this lesson, you should be able to do the following:

- Apply knowledge of current, approved ICD-10-CM coding guidelines to assign and sequence codes related to diseases of the respiratory system
- Identify the various types of respiratory disorders
- Differentiate among the various types of pneumonia
- Understand the appropriate use of status asthmaticus
- Explain the differences between alkalosis and acidosis

ICD-10-CM

Chapter 10 of the ICD-10-CM code book includes the following sections:

J00–J06	Acute upper respiratory infections
J09–J18	Influenza and pneumonia
J20–J22	Other acute lower respiratory infections
J30–J39	Other diseases of upper respiratory tract
J40–J47	Chronic lower respiratory diseases
J60–J70	Lung diseases due to external agents
J80–J84	Other respiratory diseases principally affecting the interstitium
J85–J86	Suppurative and necrotic conditions of the lower respiratory tract
J90–J94	Other diseases of the pleura
J95	Intraoperative and postprocedural complications and disorders of respiratory system, not elsewhere classified
J96–J99	Other diseases of the respiratory system

These diseases are most often treated by internists, allergists, and ear, nose, and throat doctors, also called ENT specialists or otolaryngologists.

A note appears at the beginning of Chapter 10 in the code book that instructs the coder to use an additional code, where applicable, to identify exposure to environmental tobacco smoke (Z77.22), exposure to tobacco smoke in the perinatal period (P96.81), history of tobacco use

(Z87.891), occupational exposure to environmental tobacco smoke (Z57.31), tobacco dependence (F17.-), and tobacco use (Z72.0).

Acute Upper Respiratory Infections

Upper respiratory infection (URI) is the sudden, severe onset of inflammation of an undetermined site in the airway tract above the bronchi. The following conditions are reported using these codes:

- J00   Acute nasopharyngitis (common cold)
- J01   Acute sinusitis
- J02   Acute pharyngitis
- J03   Acute tonsillitis
- J04   Acute laryngitis and tracheitis
- J05   Acute obstructive laryngitis [croup] and epiglottitis
- J06   Acute upper respiratory infections of multiple and unspecified sites

Without further specification, URI is reported with code J06.9.

Sinusitis

Sinusitis is inflammation of a sinus, particularly the paranasal sinuses (maxillary, frontal, ethmoidal, or sphenoidal). Acute sinusitis is an acute inflammation of the air-filled sinuses that contributes to blockage of the sinus openings and obstruction of their ventilation and drainage. ICD-10-CM classifies acute sinusitis, unspecified, to category J01.9, with the fourth characters identifying whether the sinusitis is recurrent or not. When the diagnosis indicates acute pansinusitis (all sinuses), code J01.40 is reported. Chronic sinusitis is a chronic inflammation of the paranasal sinuses following persistent bacterial infection. ICD-10-CM classifies chronic sinusitis to category J32.9.

Diseases of the Tonsils and Adenoids

Tonsillitis is inflammation of the tonsils and may be classified as acute or chronic. Acute tonsillitis is characterized by sore throat, fever, chills, swollen and tender submandibular lymph glands, inflamed tonsils, malaise, pain referred to ears, and purulent drainage from the tonsillar pillars. ICD-10-CM classifies acute tonsillitis to code J03. Chronic tonsillitis is characterized by recurrent attacks of acute tonsillitis, recurrent colds, unexplained fever, loss of appetite, tiredness, and a scarred, fissured appearance on the tonsillar surface. Treatment includes antibiotic therapy and tonsillectomy. When the diagnosis is identified as hypertrophy of the tonsils or adenoids, the following codes are available:

- J35.1   Hypertrophy of tonsils
- J35.2   Hypertrophy of adenoids
- J35.3   Hypertrophy of tonsils with hypertrophy of adenoids

Influenza and Pneumonia

Various types of influenza are reported with codes J09–J11. Influenza due to novel influenza A is reported with subcategory code J09.X. Fifth characters identify manifestations such as pneumonia, gastrointestinal manifestations, other respiratory manifestations, and other manifestations. Avian influenza virus is included in subcategory J09.X, as is bird influenza and swine influenza. Avian influenza is influenza infection in birds. The virus that causes the bird infection can change (mutate) to infect humans. The first avian influenza virus to infect humans occurred in Hong Kong in 1997. The epidemic was linked to chickens and classified as avian influenza A (H1N1). Outbreaks of identified H1N1 influenza virus with the accompanying complications were widely reported in 2009.

Category J09, Influenza due to certain identified influenza viruses, is further subdivided:

- J09.X Influenza due to identified novel influenza A virus

  J09.X1 Influenza due to identified novel influenza A virus with pneumonia

  J09.X2 Influenza due to identified novel influenza A virus with other respiratory manifestations

  J09.X3 Influenza due to identified novel influenza A virus with gastrointestinal manifestations

  J04.X9 Influenza due to identified novel influenza A virus with other manifestations

Category J10, Influenza due to other identified influenza virus
Category J11, Influenza due to unidentified influenza virus
Categories J10–J11 subcategories have similar structures to category J09.

Pneumonia is inflammation of the lung with exudate. It is classified by the underlying cause (bacterial, viral, protozoal, fungal, mycobacterial, mycoplasmal, or rickettsial infection) or as a result of aspiration or surgery. ICD-10-CM classifies most pneumonias to the following categories, most of which are subdivided to identify specific types or specific organisms:

- J12 Viral pneumonia, not elsewhere classified
- J13 Pneumonia due to Streptococcus pneumoniae
- J14 Pneumonia due to Hemophilus influenza
- J15 Bacterial pneumonia, not elsewhere classified
- J16 Pneumonia due to other infectious organisms, not elsewhere classified
- J17 Pneumonia in diseases classified elsewhere
- J18 Pneumonia, unspecified organism

Viral Pneumonia

Viral pneumonia (category J12) is subdivided to fourth character subcategories that identify the specific virus such as J12.0, Adenoviral pneumonia. It is a highly contagious disease affecting both the trachea and the bronchi of the lungs. Inflammation destroys the action of the cilia and causes hemorrhage. Isolation of the virus is difficult, and x-rays do not reveal any pulmonary changes.

Streptococcal Pneumonia

Streptococcus pneumoniae pneumonia (category J13) describes pneumonia caused by the pneumococcal bacteria. The bacteria lodge in the alveoli and cause an inflammation. When the pleura are involved, the irritated surfaces rub together and cause painful breathing. On examination, pleural friction can be heard. A chest x-ray demonstrates a consolidation of the lungs that results from pus forming in the alveoli and replacing the air. Approximately 90 percent of lobar pneumonia is due to pneumococcal bacteria. Bronchopneumonia usually begins in the terminal bronchioles of the lung and causes the air space to become filled with exudates.

Bacterial Pneumonia, NEC

Other bacterial pneumonia (category J15) is subdivided to fourth-digit subcategories that identify specific bacteria such as *Klebsiella pneumoniae* (J15.0), *Pseudomonas* (J15.1), *Streptococcus, Group B* (J15.3), and *Staphylococcus* (J15.2). The following codes are included in subcategory J15.2:

- J15.211 Pneumonia due to Methicillin susceptible Staphylococcus aureus
- J15.212 Pneumonia due to Methicillin resistant Staphylococcus aureus

Bacteria are the most common cause of pneumonia in adults. Gram staining is a rapid and cost-effective method for diagnosing bacterial pneumonia when a good sputum sample is available. Gram-negative pneumonia, NEC, is classified as J15.6. Pneumonia due to gram-positive bacteria is coded to J15.9.

Pneumonia in Infectious Diseases Classified Elsewhere

Pneumonia in infectious diseases classified elsewhere (category J17) is set in italic type and thus is not meant for primary tabulation. In addition, instructional notations in this category direct coders to code first the underlying disease.

Pneumonia, Unspecified Organism

Category J18.9, Pneumonia, unspecified organism, is a fourth character that should be assigned only when the health record does not identify the causative organism.

Ventilator-Associated Pneumonia (VAP)

Code J95.851 is used when a diagnosis of ventilator-associated pneumonia (VAP) is made. The diagnosis of VAP can be made only by the physician. The specific organism, if known, should be assigned as well. It is not necessary to assign a code from J12 through J18 to identify the specific type of pneumonia, unless the patient is admitted with one type of pneumonia and subsequently develops VAP. The Excludes statement indicates that ventilator lung in newborn is reported with P27.8.

Aspiration Pneumonitis

Category J69, Pneumonitis due to solids and liquids, is subdivided to fourth-character subcategories that describe the causative agent. This category is also referred to as aspiration pneumonia. When the causative agent is unspecified, the Alphabetic Index offers direction to code J69.8. In cases where the patient develops both aspiration pneumonia and bacterial pneumonia, codes for both types of pneumonia should be assigned.

Acute Bronchitis

Bronchitis is an inflammation of the bronchi and can be acute or chronic in nature. Acute bronchitis involves the tracheobronchial tree and is often due to exposure to cold, inhalation of irritating substances, or acute infections. ICD-10-CM classifies acute bronchitis to code J20, which includes the following diagnoses:

- J20.0   Acute bronchitis due to Mycoplasma pneumoniae
- J20.1   Acute bronchitis due to Hemophilus influenzae
- J20.2   Acute bronchitis due to streptococcus
- J20.3   Acute bronchitis due to coxsackievirus
- J20.4   Acute bronchitis due to parainfluenza virus
- J20.5   Acute bronchitis due to respiratory syncytial virus
- J20.6   Acute bronchitis due to rhinovirus
- J20.7   Acute bronchitis due to echovirus
- J20.8   Acute bronchitis due to other specified organisms
- J20.9   Acute bronchitis, unspecified

Chronic Lower Respiratory Disease

Conditions of the lower respiratory systems may be treated on both the inpatient and outpatient basis. Some of the more common conditions are listed below.

Chronic Bronchitis

ICD-10-CM classifies chronic bronchitis to category J42 and includes chronic bronchitis NOS, chronic tracheitis, and chronic tracheobronchitis. When bronchitis is described as simple and mucopurulent, code J41 is assigned. When a diagnosis of bronchitis is given with no indication of chronic or acute, code J40 is reported. When bronchitis is associated with chronic obstructive pulmonary disease (COPD), a code from J44 should be reported. Chronic bronchitis is associated with prolonged exposure to nonspecific bronchial irritants and accompanied by mucous hypersecretion and certain structural changes in the bronchi. Usually associated with cigarette smoking, one form of bronchitis is characterized clinically by a chronic productive cough.

Emphysema

Emphysema is a lung disease that reduces the ability of the lungs to expel air because of damage to the bronchioles. A person with emphysema may be short of breath initially during exertion, but, as the disease progresses, even during rest.

ICD-10-CM code J43 is used to report emphysema. The following four character codes are used to report emphysema:

- J43.0   Unilateral plumonary emphysema [MacLeod's syndrome]
- J43.1   Panlobular emphysema
- J43.2   Centrilobular emphysema
- J43.8   Other emphysema
- J43.9   Emphysema, unspecified

Chronic Obstructive Pulmonary Disease

COPD is characterized by the decreased ability of the lungs to perform ventilation due to diffuse obstruction of the smaller bronchi and bronchioles, which results in coughing, wheezing, shortness of breath, and disturbances of gas exchange (O_2 and CO_2). Exacerbations of COPD, such as episodes of increased shortness of breath and cough, are often treated on an outpatient basis. More severe exacerbations, such as pneumonia, bronchitis, or other infections, usually result in admission to the hospital.

Treatment consists of oxygen support, arterial blood gas (ABG) monitoring, intravenous or aerosol medication, and chest physical therapy as well as possible intubation with mechanical ventilation or tracheostomy. Medications frequently prescribed include inhaled bronchodilators (Alupent, Proventil, Ventolin, Atrovent) or oral bronchodilators (theophylline, albuterol).

The clinical course of COPD is extremely varied. However, two patterns of symptoms are often superimposed on each other: a progressive worsening of underlying lung function (progressive dyspnea, fatigue, and exacerbations) with recurring URIs or lung infections. Stress caused by congestive heart failure (CHF) may lead to rapid deterioration of COPD.

COPD is classified to code J44. The various types of diagnoses included are as follows:

- J44.0   Chronic obstructive pulmonary disease with acute lower respiratory infection
- J44.1   Chronic obstructive pulmonary disease with (acute) exacerbation
- J44.9   Chronic obstructive pulmonary disease, unspecified

Asthma

Asthma is characterized by difficult and labored breathing with coughing and wheezing due to spasmodic contraction of the bronchi or inflammation of the mucous membrane lining of the bronchi. In some cases, it is an allergic manifestation in sensitized persons. The term *reactive airway disease* (RAD) is considered synonymous with asthma. Asthma is reported with category J45. Fourth digit codes identify the type of asthma, and fifth digits indicate the presence of status asthmaticus or acute exacerbation. When describing asthma, the terminology has been updated to reflect the clinical classification of asthma. For example, the term *mild intermittent* must be clarified with one of three degrees of persistence: mild persistent, moderate persistent, and severe persistent.

Status asthmaticus is an acute asthmatic attack in which the degree of bronchial obstruction is not relieved by usual treatments, such as epinephrine or aminophylline. Other terms that may be used to describe status asthmaticus include *intractable asthmatic attack*, *refractory asthma*, *severe prolonged asthmatic attack*, *airway obstruction not relieved by bronchodilators*, and *severe intractable wheezing*. Status asthmaticus is assigned only when there is specific documentation by the physician. When the coder suspects status asthmaticus based on the descriptors above, the coder should query the physician. When both acute exacerbation and status asthmaticus are used by the physician, only the status asthmaticus is coded.

The coder should review the Excludes 1 and Excludes 2 statements under J45.

Bronchospasm

Acute bronchospasm is an integral part of chronic airway obstruction and is not coded separately. However, when an underlying cause is not specified, code J98.01 is reported.

Pleural Effusion

Pleural effusion is inflammation of the visceral and parietal layers of the pleural cavity. Pain develops when the visceral layer lining the lungs expands with breathing and moves over and irritates the inflamed sensory nerve endings in the fixed parietal layer lining the thoracic cavity. Common causes of pleural effusion include pneumonia, tuberculosis, pneumothorax, viral infection, pulmonary embolism, malignant process, lung abscess, systemic lupus erythematosus, bronchiectasis, rheumatoid arthritis, and pulmonary infarction. Codes for pleurisy may be found in a variety of places. For example, malignant pleural effusion is reported with code J91.0. The coder is instructed to "Code first the underlying neoplasm." Tuberculous effusion is reported with code A15.6. Without further specification, pleural effusion is reported with code J90.

Adult Pulmonary Langerhans' Cell Histiocytosis (PLCH)

Adult PLCH is a rare interstitial lung disease of unknown etiology that occurs almost exclusively in smokers. In adults, pulmonary involvement with Langerhans' cell histiocytosis usually occurs as a single-system disease and is characterized by focal Langerhans' cell granulomas infiltrating and destroying distal bronchioles. Code J84.82 identifies Adult PLCH.

Interstitial Lung Diseases of Childhood

There are a number of interstitial lung diseases that affect children. These include code J84.841, neuroendrocrine cell hyperplasia of infancy (NEHI), pulmonary interstitial glycogenosis (J84.842), and code J84.843 for alveolar capillary dysplasia with vein misalignment (ACD/MPV).

Other Alveolar and Parietoalveolar Pneumonopathy

There are a variety of idiopathic interstitial pneumonopathies, a group of scarring lung diseases with distinctive presentations, pathophysiology, and clinical course. These conditions are classified to category J84.0. Fifth characters are used to report the following:

- J84.01   Alveolar proteinosis
- J84.02   Pulmonary alveolar microlithiasis
- J84.03   Idiopathic pulmonary hemosiderosis
- J84.09   Other alveolar and parieto-alveolar conditions

Pneumothorax

Pneumothorax is the abnormal accumulation of air or gas in the space separating the visceral and parietal pleural layers. There are several types of pneumothorax, including spontaneous, iatrogenic, or traumatic. Spontaneous tension pneumothorax is characterized by the ability of air to enter the pleural space, but the inability for it to escape. Iatrogenic pneumothorax, also known as postoperative pneumothorax, occurs as a result of surgical treatment or other medical care. Traumatic pneumothorax occurs as a result of trauma and may involve either an open or a closed chest wound. ICD-10-CM classifies most types of pneumothorax and air leak to category J93, which is further subdivided to specify the type, such as spontaneous tension (J93.0). Without further specification, pneumothorax is reported with code J93.9, Pneumothorax, unspecified. Traumatic pneumothorax is reported with code S27.0XXA.

Respiratory Failure and Insufficiency

Respiratory failure is the inability of the respiratory system to supply adequate oxygen to maintain proper metabolism or eliminate carbon dioxide. Respiratory failure is classified into four categories:

- J96.0   Acute respiratory failure
- J96.1   Chronic respiratory failure
- J96.2   Acute and chronic respiratory failure
- J96.9   Respiratory failure, unspecified

Fifth characters identify the presence of hypoxia, hypercapnia, or both.

Respiratory failure is assigned when documentation in the health record supports its use. It may be due to, or associated with, other respiratory conditions, such as pneumonia, chronic bronchitis, or COPD. Respiratory failure also may be due to, or associated with, nonrespiratory conditions, such as myasthenia gravis, CHF, myocardial infarction (MI), or cerebrovascular accident (CVA).

Acute respiratory distress syndrome (ARDS) is a life-threatening condition that involves very low oxygen levels in the blood. It is often seen as a result of injury, blood transfusion, aspiration, or drug or alcohol use. ARDS is coded with J80, Acute respiratory distress syndrome.

Other types of abnormalities of breathing with no established diagnosis are coded to category R06, Abnormalities of breathing.

Guidelines for Coding and Sequencing of Respiratory Failure

1. Acute respiratory failure (J96.00) may be assigned as the principal or first-listed diagnosis when it is the condition established after study to be chiefly responsible for occasioning the admission to the hospital, and the selection is supported by the Alphabetic Index and Tabular List. However, chapter-specific guidelines (obstetrics, poisoning, HIV, newborn) that provide sequencing direction take precedence.

2. Respiratory failure may be listed as a secondary diagnosis if it occurs after admission or is present on admission but does not meet the definition of principal diagnosis.

3. When a patient is admitted with respiratory failure and another acute condition (for example, MI or CVA), the principal diagnosis will not be the same in every situation. Selection of the principal diagnosis will be dependent on the circumstances of the admission. If both the respiratory failure and the other acute condition are responsible for occasioning the admission to the hospital, the guideline regarding two or more diagnoses that equally meet the definition for principal diagnosis should be applied. If the documentation is not clear as to whether acute respiratory failure and another condition are equally responsible for occasioning the admission, query the provider for clarification.

Some examples of selecting the first-listed diagnosis include the following:

EXAMPLE 1: A patient with chronic myasthenia gravis suffers an acute exacerbation and develops acute respiratory failure. The patient is admitted to the hospital in respiratory failure.

First-listed: J96.00   Acute respiratory failure

Additional: G70.01   Myasthenia gravis with (acute) exacerbation

EXAMPLE 2: A patient with emphysema develops acute respiratory failure. The patient is admitted to the hospital for treatment of respiratory failure.

First-listed: J96.00   Acute respiratory failure

Additional: J43.9   Emphysema

EXAMPLE 3: A patient with congestive heart failure is brought to the emergency department in acute respiratory failure. The patient is admitted, and the physician documents that acute respiratory failure is the reason for admission.

First-listed: J96.00   Acute respiratory failure

Additional: I50.9   Congestive heart failure

EXAMPLE 4: A patient is admitted with respiratory failure due to *Pneumocystis carinii* pneumonia, which is associated with AIDS.

First-listed: B20   Human immunodeficiency virus (HIV) disease

Additional: J96.00   Acute respiratory failure

B59   Pneumocystosis

Pulmonary Edema

Pulmonary edema is an abnormal, diffuse accumulation of fluid in the tissues and alveolar spaces of the lung that is characterized clinically by dyspnea and, when severe, by cyanosis. For classification purposes, pulmonary edema can be described as acute pulmonary edema of cardiac origin, acute pulmonary edema of noncardiac origin, or chronic pulmonary edema.

Acute Pulmonary Edema of Cardiac Origin

Because this condition is a manifestation of heart failure, use codes from Chapter 9, Diseases of the circulatory system (I00–I99). Documentation in the health record of a patient with acute pulmonary edema of cardiogenic origin usually references cardiac enlargement, presence of S3 gallop, elevated pulmonary artery wedge pressure, or associated cardiac diseases. Frequently, the chest x-ray will show pleural effusions. Treatment often includes diuretics and other cardiac medications. For example, pulmonary edema in conjunction with left ventricular failure is included in code I50.1. However, pulmonary edema in conjunction with ischemic heart diseases, including acute MI or acute ischemic heart disease, is coded separately.

Acute Pulmonary Edema of Noncardiac Origin

Other forms of acute pulmonary edema that are noncardiogenic in origin are classified to diseases of the lung or to trauma. Some examples are as follows:

- J70.0   Acute pulmonary manifestations due to radiation
- J81.0   Acute pulmonary edema
- J68.1   Pulmonary edema due to chemicals, gases, fumes, and vapors

Chronic Pulmonary Edema

Chronic pulmonary edema or pulmonary edema not otherwise specified (NOS) that is not of cardiogenic origin is coded to J81.1, Chronic pulmonary edema. But the health record or the physician should be consulted for further information to ensure that the pulmonary edema was not actually the acute type.

Alkalosis Versus Acidosis

Assessments of ABG results are performed to determine whether respiratory acidosis or alkalosis or metabolic acidosis has developed. Key components of ABGs, which are interpreted by the clinician, are the oxygen level (pO_2), the acid-base balance (pH), the buffer level of bicarbonate ions (HCO_3), and the oxyhemoglobin saturation (O_2) in the blood.

The traditional method of interpreting the acid-base status of ABGs uses the terminology *uncompensated*, *partially compensated*, and *compensated*, along with the normal ranges for pCO_2 and pH. Table 11.1 lists the values for pH, pCO_2, and HCO_3 for both respiratory acidosis and alkalosis and metabolic acidosis and alkalosis.

Table 11.1. Values for acidosis and alkalosis

Status	pH	pCO_2	HCO_2
Respiratory Acidosis			
Uncompensated	<7.35	>45	normal
Partially compensated	<7.35	>45	>27
Compensated	7.35–7.45	>45	>27
Respiratory Alkalosis			
Uncompensated	>7.45	<35	normal
Partially compensated	>7.45	<35	<22
Compensated	7.40–7.45	<35	<22
Metabolic Acidosis			
Uncompensated	<7.35	normal	<22
Partially compensated	<7.35	<35	<22

Continued

Table 11.1.   Values for acidosis and alkalosis (continued)

Status	pH	pCO$_2$	HCO$_2$
Compensated	7.35–7.40	<35	<22
Metabolic Alkalosis			
Uncompensated	>7.45	normal	>27
Partially compensated*	>7.45	>45	>27
Compensated**	7.40–7.45	>45	>27

*Partially compensated and **compensated metabolic alkalosis occur infrequently because of the body's mechanism to prevent hypoventilation.

Causes of respiratory acidosis or primary hypercapnia (increase in CO$_2$) include the following:

- Cardiopulmonary disease (specifically asthma with status asthmaticus)
- Severe bilateral pneumonia or bronchopneumonia
- Severe pulmonary edema
- COPD (bronchitis, bronchiectasis, bronchiolitis, emphysema)
- Interstitial fibrosis
- Severe chronic pneumonitis
- Central nervous system depression by drugs, trauma, or lesion
- Neurologic or neuromuscular disease resulting in weakness of respiratory muscles
- Fatigue following any acute lung disease

Clinical manifestations of respiratory acidosis include irritability, headache, mental cloudiness, apathy, confusion, incoherence, combativeness, hallucinations, and cardiac arrhythmias.

Causes of respiratory alkalosis or primary hypocapnia (reduction in CO$_2$) include the following:

- Compensation for primary metabolic acidosis
- Pneumonia
- Pulmonary edema
- Asthma
- Pneumothorax
- Pulmonary fibrosis
- Drugs such as doxapram, salicylates, and progesterone
- Nicotinic hepatic failure
- Sepsis

Symptoms of respiratory alkalosis include light-headedness and confusion.

Primary causes of metabolic acidosis are ketoacidosis, renal failure, and ingestion of base-depleting drugs such as alcohol and aspirin. Causes of metabolic alkalosis are hypokalemia, gastric vomiting or suctioning, massive doses of steroids, and diuretics.

The following ICD-10-CM codes are for classifying these conditions:

- E87.2   Acidosis
- E87.3   Alkalosis

Z Codes Related to the Respiratory System

Subcategory Z99 is used to demonstrate dependence on a respirator or ventilator.

- Z99.0   Dependence on aspirator
- Z99.1   Dependence on respirator
- Z99.11   Dependence on respirator (ventilator) status
- Z99.12   Encounter for respirator (ventilator) dependence during power failure

Chapter 11: ICD-10-CM Exercises

Review the following statements and cases and assign the appropriate codes:

1. Obstructive chronic bronchitis

2. Chronic maxillary sinusitis

3. Severe persistent asthma with status asthmaticus

4. Pneumococcal pleural effusion

5. Acute upper respiratory infection with flu

6. Acute adult respiratory distress syndrome

7. MRSA bronchopneumonia

8. Allergic pneumonitis due to wood dust

9. Pneumonia in cytomegalic inclusion disease

10. Acute and chronic respiratory failure with chronic obstructive bronchitis

11. Pneumococcal pneumonia due to HIV infection/AIDS

12. Pansinusitis with hypertrophy of nasal turbinates

13. An 84-year-old woman was transferred from the nursing home on the day of admission. She has had a persistent left upper lobe pneumonia and has received oral antibiotics for the past two weeks. The patient has become increasingly dehydrated with a persistent productive cough, which is the reason she has been admitted today. Her past medical history is also significant for chronic atrial fibrillation. A review of the chest x-rays demonstrates a fairly stable left upper lobe infiltrate with no pleural effusion. The patient seemed to improve on
Continued

intravenous (IV) fluids and IV antibiotics. She is now afebrile with clearing of the pneumonia, so she is being discharged.

Discharge diagnoses: Left upper lobe pneumonia; dehydration; chronic atrial fibrillation

14. A 67-year-old woman presented to the emergency department with a gradual increase in shortness of breath that was unresponsive to home nebulizer treatments. In the emergency department, she received more respiratory treatments, but her airway failed to clear, and she was therefore admitted to the hospital. A chest x-ray showed no evidence of active infiltrates. After being admitted, the patient received IV steroids and frequent respiratory therapy treatments. She gradually cleared and was discharged on aminophylline by mouth and Ventolin treatments, and her prednisone was reduced to 10 mg.

Discharge diagnoses: Status asthmaticus; COPD

15. Patient has acute laryngitis with airway obstruction.

16. Methicillin resistant pneumonia due to Staphylococcus aureus

17. Influenza due to identified novel influenza A virus with pneumonia

18. Postoperative pneumothorax

19. Radiation pneumonitis caused by a radioactive isotope

20. Patient was diagnosed with respiratory bronchiolitis interstitial lung disease.

21. A patient presents with an exacerbation of myasthenia gravis, which resulted in acute respiratory failure.

22. A child is seen in her pediatrician's office for hypertrophic tonsillitis with adenoiditis.

23. A patient is evaluated for allergic rhinitis and a deviated nasal septum.

24. Acute respiratory failure, acute bronchitis with acute exacerbation of COPD

25. Patient presents with the following diagnosis: Congestive heart failure with pleural effusion diagnosed by diagnostic thoracentesis.

26. A patient is seen at the walk-in clinic and diagnosed with acute asthmatic bronchitis.

27. Moderate persistent asthma with status asthmaticus. Acute exacerbation of chronic obstructive pulmonary disease.

28. The patient has aspiration pneumonia because of his difficulty in swallowing (neurogenic) due to a previous cerebral infarction. The patient also has stage 1 decubitus ulcers on both his left and right hip.

Diseases of the Digestive System

After completing this lesson, you should be able to do the following:

- Apply knowledge of current, approved ICD-10-CM coding guidelines to assign and sequence accurate codes related to diseases of the digestive system
- Identify the major types of digestive disorders

ICD-10-CM

Chapter 11 of the ICD-10-CM code book classifies diseases of the digestive system, including angiodysplasia, cholelithiasis, hernia, hepatitis, gastritis, and ulcer. The chapter is divided into the following blocks:

K00–K14	Diseases of oral cavity and salivary glands
K20–K31	Diseases of esophagus, stomach, and duodenum
K35–K38	Diseases of appendix
K40–K46	Hernia
K50–K52	Noninfective enteritis and colitis
K55–K64	Other diseases of intestines
K65–K68	Diseases of peritoneum and retroperitoneum
K70–K77	Diseases of liver
K80–K87	Disorders of gallbladder, biliary tract, and pancreas
K90–K95	Other diseases of digestive system

The diseases described in Chapter 11 are treated primarily by dentists, gastroenterologists, internists, and proctologists.

Diseases of Oral Cavity and Salivary Glands

The need for dental codes has become urgent with the advent of electronic health records and the desire of dentists to track patient conditions with their outcomes. The category codes within this section include the following:

- K00   Disorders of tooth development and eruption
- K01   Embedded and impacted teeth
- K02   Dental caries
- K03   Other diseases of hard tissues of teeth
- K04   Diseases of pulp and periapical tissues
- K05   Gingivitis and periodontal diseases
- K06   Other disorders of gingiva and edentulous alveolar ridge
- K08   Other disorders of teeth and supporting structures
- K09   Cysts of oral region, NEC
- K11   Diseases of the salivary glands
- K12   Stomatitis and related lesions
- K13   Other diseases of lip and oral mucosa
- K14   Diseases of the tongue

Additional characters under each of these provide greater specificity.

Esophagitis

Esophagitis is an inflammation of the esophageal lining. Underlying causes include the following:

- Infection
- Irritation from a nasogastric (NG) tube
- Backflow of gastric juice from the stomach (most common cause)

ICD-10-CM classifies esophagitis to subcategory K20, with a fourth character to describe the specific type. The code book reminds coders to assign an additional code to identify alcohol use and dependence. Subcategory K22.1, Ulcer of esophagus, has been expanded to include the following codes:

- K22.10   Ulcer of esophagus without bleeding
- K22.11   Ulcer of esophagus with bleeding

Barrett's esophagus is identified by code K22.7, with fifth and sixth characters identifying the presence (and grade) or absence of dysplasia.

Complications of Esophagostomy

Complications of esophagostomy are identified using codes K94.3, Esophagostomy complications. Fifth characters identify hemorrhage, infection, or malfunction.

Gastrointestinal Ulcers

Ulcers of the gastrointestinal (GI) tract are characterized by an inflammatory, necrotic, sloughing defect. ICD-10-CM classifies these ulcers to categories K25–K28, which further subdivide to indicate severity (acute versus chronic) and associated complications, such as hemorrhage, perforation, or hemorrhage and perforation. The categories classifying GI ulcers include the following:

- K25   Gastric ulcer
- K26   Duodenal ulcer
- K27   Peptic ulcer, site unspecified
- K28   Gastrojejunal ulcer

The preceding categories are subdivided to fourth character subcategories that describe acute and chronic conditions and the presence of hemorrhage or perforation.

The bleeding ulcer or hemorrhage does not have to be actively bleeding at the time of the examination in order to use the code for ulcer with hemorrhage. A statement by the physician that bleeding has occurred and that it is attributed to the ulcer is sufficient.

Complications of Weight Loss Procedures

Bariatric surgery and gastric band procedures have some associated risks such as infections and device malfunctions. Complications of bariatric surgery are indexed to code K95, Complications of bariatric surgery. Appropriate codes are as follows:

- K95.0   Complications of gastric band procedure

    K95.01   Infection due to gastric band procedure
    K95.09   Other complications of gastric band procedure

- K95.8   Complications of other bariatric procedure

    K95.81   Infections due to other bariatric procedure
    K95.89   Other complications of other bariatric procedure

The coder should review the several "use additional code" notes under these codes.

Diverticular Disease

A diverticulum of the intestine is a mucosal pouch, or sac, that herniates through a defect in the muscular layer of the intestinal wall. ICD-10-CM classifies diverticula to category K57, with a fourth character to identify the specific site (with or without perforation or abscess) and a fifth character to indicate the presence or absence of hemorrhage and the progression of the disease (diverticulosis versus diverticulitis). Diverticulosis is the presence of diverticula in the intestines, especially in the large intestine. It also results from herniation of the mucosa through defects in the muscular wall, usually at the site of blood vessel entry. Diverticulitis is the inflammation and infection of a diverticulum.

Diverticula are reported as either acquired or congenital. For certain sites, ICD-10-CM assumes that the condition is congenital (unless otherwise reported), whereas for other sites, the assumption is that the diverticula are acquired. An example of the Alphabetic Index under diverticulum, diverticula, is shown below:

> **EXAMPLE**:   Diverticulum, diverticula
>
> Esophagus (congenital)

Therefore, unless the physician directs otherwise, diverticula of the esophagus are considered congenital.

Eosinophilic Gastrointestinal Disorders

Eosinophilic gastrointestinal disorders (EGIDs) involve eosinophil accumulations in the tissue lining the gastrointestinal tract, in the absence of known causes for eosinophilia, such as drug reactions, parasitic infection, connective tissue disease, or malignancy.

The EGIDs include eosinophilic esophagitis (K20.0), eosinophilic gastritis (K52.81), eosinophilic gastroenteritis (K52.81), and eosinophilic colitis (K52.82).

Appendicitis

Acute appendicitis (category K35) is inflammation of the appendix, with the onset being sudden and severe. It is a very common disease requiring major surgery. Appendicitis begins with generalized or localized abdominal pain in the upper right abdomen, followed by anorexia, nausea, and vomiting. The pain eventually localizes in the lower right abdomen with abdominal board-like rigidity, retractive respirations, increasing tenderness, and increasingly severe abdominal spasm. Appendectomy is the only effective treatment.

ICD-10-CM classifies appendicitis with generalized peritonitis to code K35.2. Acute appendicitis with localized peritonitis is reported with K35.3.

Appendicitis described as chronic or recurrent is coded to K36, Other appendicitis. Unspecified appendicitis is reported with code K37.

Hernias

Hernias of the abdominal cavity are classified to categories K40 through K46. A fifth character is used to describe whether the hernia is unilateral, bilateral, or with an additional complication (gangrene or obstruction).

A hernia is the protrusion of a loop or knuckle of an organ or a tissue through an abdominal opening. Many different types of hernias exist, including the following:

- An inguinal hernia is a hernia of an intestinal loop into the inguinal canal.

- A femoral hernia is a hernia of a loop of intestine into the femoral canal.

- A hiatal hernia is the displacement of the upper part of the stomach into the thorax through the esophageal opening (hiatus) of the diaphragm.

- A diaphragmatic hernia is the protrusion of an abdominal organ into the chest cavity through a defect in the diaphragm.

- A ventral hernia, or an abdominal hernia, is a herniation of the intestine or some other internal body structure through the abdominal wall.

- An incisional hernia is an abdominal hernia at the site of a previously made incision.

- An umbilical hernia is a type of abdominal hernia, in which part of the intestine protrudes at the umbilicus and is covered by skin and subcutaneous tissue. This type may also be described as an omphalocele.

ICD-10-CM uses the term *obstruction* to indicate that incarceration, irreducibility, or strangulation is present with the hernia. A hernia with both obstruction and gangrene is classified as hernia with gangrene.

- An irreducible hernia is also known as an incarcerated hernia. An incarcerated hernia is a hernia of the intestine that cannot be returned or reduced by manipulation; it may be strangulated.

- A strangulated hernia is an incarcerated hernia that is so tightly constricted as to restrict the blood supply to the contents of the hernial sac and possibly cause gangrene of the contents, such as the intestine. This represents a medical emergency requiring surgical correction.

Codes for different types of hernias of the abdominal cavity are included in the following categories:

- K40   Inguinal hernia
- K41   Femoral hernia
    - K42   Umbilical hernia
    - K43   Ventral hernia
    - K44   Diaphragmatic hernia
    - K45   Other abdominal hernia
    - K46   Specified abdominal hernia

Fourth and fifth characters add specificity:

- K41.0   Bilateral femoral hernia, with obstruction, without gangrene
    - K41.00   Bilateral femoral hernia, with obstruction, without gangrene, not specified as recurrent
    - K41.01   Bilateral femoral hernia, with obstruction, without gangrene, recurrent
- K41.1   Bilateral femoral hernia, with gangrene
    - K41.10   Bilateral femoral hernia, with gangrene, not specified as recurrent
    - K41.11   Bilateral femoral hernia, with gangrene, recurrent
- K41.4   Unilateral femoral hernia, with gangrene
    - K41.40   Unilateral femoral hernia, with gangrene, not specified as recurrent
    - K41.41   Unilateral femoral hernia, with gangrene, recurrent

Crohn's Disease

Regional enteritis, also known as Crohn's disease or granulomatous enteritis, is a chronic inflammatory disease commonly affecting the distal ileum and colon. It is characterized by chronic diarrhea, abdominal pain, fever, anorexia, weight loss, right lower quadrant mass or fullness, and lymphadenitis of the mesenteric nodes. ICD-10-CM classifies regional enteritis to category K50, with the fourth character digit identifying the specific site affected (for example, the large intestine) and the fifth and sixth characters identifying complications of Crohn's disease. Some examples of codes from category K50 include:

- K50.0   Crohn's disease of small intestine
    - K50.00   Crohn's disease of small intestine without complications
    - K50.01   Crohn's disease of small intestine with complications
        - K50.011   Crohn's disease of small intestine with rectal bleeding
        - K50.012   Crohn's disease of small intestine with intestinal obstruction
        - K50.013   Crohn's disease of small intestine with fistula
        - K50.014   Crohn's disease of small intestine with abscess
        - K50.018   Crohn's disease of small intestine with other complication
        - K50.019   Crohn's disease of small intestine with unspecified complications

Gastroenteritis

Gastroenteritis is an inflammation of the stomach, small intestine, or colon. It is characterized by diarrhea, nausea and vomiting, and abdominal cramps. Gastroenteritis can be caused by bacteria, amoebae, parasites, viruses, ingestion of toxins, drug reactions, enzyme deficiencies, or food allergens. ICD-10-CM classifies gastroenteritis according to the cause:

- A02.0   Salmonella enteritis
- K52.2   Allergic and dietetic gastroenteritis and colitis
- K52.1   Toxic gastroenteritis and colitis

Without further specification as to site of gastroenteritis, code K52.9 should be assigned. When coding infectious gastroenteritis, the coder is referred to Enteritis, infectious. Note that gastroenteritis due to an infectious process is classified to Chapter 1 of the ICD-10-CM code book, Infectious and parasitic diseases. These codes are based on the infecting organism, such as *Clostridium difficile*, A04.7.

Gastritis and Duodenitis

Gastritis is inflammation of the gastric mucosa and may be described as acute or chronic. ICD-10-CM classifies gastritis to category K29, which further subdivides at the fourth character level to identify the underlying cause or specific type, with the fifth character indicating the presence or absence of hemorrhage. The subcategories include the following:

- K29.0   Acute gastritis

  K29.2   Alcoholic gastritis
  K29.3   Chronic superficial gastritis
  K29.4   Chronic atrophic gastritis
  K29.5   Unspecified chronic gastritis
  K29.6   Other gastritis
  K29.7   Gastritis, unspecified
  K29.8   Duodenitis
  K29.9   Gastroduodenitis, unspecified

Active bleeding during the current examination or procedure does not have to be present to use the fifth character to describe the hemorrhage. It may be diagnosed clinically by the physician.

Enterostomy Complications

A colostomy is a surgically created opening (stoma) between the colon and the abdominal wall. An enterostomy is a surgically created opening between other parts of the intestines and the abdominal wall. Complications of a colostomy or an enterostomy are classified to subcategory K94, Complications of artificial openings of the digestive system, which is further subdivided as follows:

- K94.0   Colostomy complication, unspecified
- K94.1   Enterostomy complication
- K94.2   Gastrostomy complications
- K94.3   Esophagostomy complications

Fifth characters identify hemorrhage, infection, or malfunction. When coding infections, the coder also should assign a code to identify the underlying organism, such as *Staphylococcus aureus*. An additional code should be used to specify the type of infection, such as sepsis.

Pouchitis

Pouchitis is a nonspecific inflammation of an internal ileoanal pouch that has been created following the removal of part of the colon. The surgical procedure is a restorative proctocolectomy with ilial pouch anal anastomosis, and it may be done for the treatment of ulcerative colitis or familial adenomatous polyposis. Creation of the pouch takes the place of a permanent ileostomy.

Symptoms of pouchitis include diarrhea, urgency, and incontinence. These may be accompanied by abdominal pain, fever, and loss of appetite.

Subcategory K91.85, Complications of intestinal pouch, is subdivided as follows:

- K91.850, Pouchitis
- K91.858, Other complications of intestinal pouch

Anal Fissure and Fistula

An anal fistula is an opening at or near the anus, usually (but not always) into the rectum above the internal sphincter. An anal fissure is a crack or slit in the mucous membrane of the anus. Fissures are very painful and difficult to heal. ICD-10-CM classifies these conditions to category as follows:

- K60.0   Acute anal fissure
- K60.1   Chronic anal fistula
- K60.2   Anal fissure, unspecified
- K60.3   Anal fistula
- K60.4   Rectal fistula
- K60.5   Anorectal fistula

Fibrosis and Cirrhosis of Liver

Cirrhosis of the liver, a long-term condition characterized by a fiber-like tissue covering the liver, results in a breakdown of the liver tissue and subsequent replacement by fat. ICD-10-CM classifies liver cirrhosis to category K74, which further subdivides to identify specific types of liver conditions such as fibrosis, sclerosis, and cirrhosis. The coder is instructed to "Code also" viral hepatitis (acute) (chronic) if applicable. Careful review of the Excludes 1 statement shows that several conditions related to the liver would be classified elsewhere. For example, alcoholic cirrhosis of the liver is reported with K70.3.

Hemorrhage of the Digestive Tract

Gastrointestinal (GI) hemorrhage is the abnormal escape of blood from the GI tract. Some common causes of upper GI bleeding include duodenal ulcer, gastric or duodenal erosions, varices, and gastric ulcer. Common causes of lower GI bleeding include diverticular disease, carcinoma of the colon, colon polyps, inflammatory bowel disease (ulcerative colitis, Crohn's disease), and angiodysplasia. The presentation of GI bleeding can vary from that of occult bleeding to acute hemorrhage. Upper GI bleeding may be identified when the patient vomits bright red blood or by the analysis of gastric fluid obtained through the NG tube. Lower GI bleeding may be identified by the asymptomatic passage of maroon-colored stool or bright red blood. The bleeding may be brisk and intermittent over several days. ICD-10-CM classifies GI hemorrhage to category K92, which further subdivides to identify the specific site of the bleeding, as follows:

- K92.0   Hematemesis (vomiting of blood)
- K92.1   Melena (bloody stool)
- K92.2   Gastrointestinal hemorrhage, unspecified

The coder should carefully review the extensive Excludes statement under category K92.2. Hemorrhage due to a specific cause or from a specific site is excluded from K92.2. For example, acute hemorrhagic gastritis is reported with code K29.01.

A positive occult blood test without further specification as to cause is reported with code R19.5, Other fecal abnormalities.

Peritonitis and Retroperitoneal Infections

Peritonitis is inflammation of the peritoneum, usually accompanied by abdominal pain and tenderness, constipation, vomiting, and moderate fever. It may be caused by a bacteria, such as *Staphylococcus*, *Pseudomonas*, or *Mycobacterium*; it may be fungal, most commonly *Candida* peritonitis, or caused by other factors, such as trauma or childbirth.

Category K65, Peritonitis, is often used with other digestive system codes. Fourth characters identify the specific type of condition:

- K65.0   Generalized (acute) peritonitis
- K65.1   Peritoneal abscess
- K65.2   Spontaneous bacterial peritonitis
- K65.3   Choleperitonitis
- K65.4   Sclerosing mesenteritis
- K65.8   Other peritonitis
- K65.9   Peritonitis, unspecified

The coder is reminded to use an additional code to identify the infectious agent, if known.

Cholecystitis and Cholelithiasis

Cholecystitis is an acute or chronic inflammation of the gallbladder. Cholelithiasis refers to gallstones in the gallbladder. Code K81 is used to report cholecystitis, with fourth characters identifying whether the condition is acute, chronic, or acute and chronic. Code K80 is used to report cholelithiasis. Fourth characters identify concurrent conditions, such as the following:

- K80.0   Calculus of gallbladder with acute cholecystitis
- K80.1   Calculus of gallbladder with other cholecystitis
- K80.2   Calculus of gallbladder without cholecystitis
- K80.3   Calculus of bile duct with cholangitis
- K80.4   Calculus of bile duct with cholecystitis
- K80.5   Calculus of bile duct without cholangitis or cholecystitis
- K80.6   Calculus of gallbladder and bile duct with cholecystitis
- K80.7   Calculus of gallbladder and bile duct without cholecystitis
- K80.0   Other cholelithiasis

A careful review of the Alphabetic Index is important in finding the appropriate codes.

Chapter 12: ICD-10-CM Exercises

Review the following statements and cases and assign the appropriate codes:

1. Reflux esophagitis

2. Hemorrhagic alcoholic gastritis

3. Diverticulosis of colon with bleeding

4. Hiatal hernia

5. Acute gastroenteritis

6. Alcoholic cirrhosis of liver

7. Chronic pancreatitis

8. Blood in stool

9. Acute perforated peptic ulcer

10. Acute appendicitis with perforation and peritoneal abscess

11. Acute cholecystitis with cholelithiasis

12. Diverticulosis and diverticulitis of colon

13. Alcoholic gastritis with hemorrhage

14. Incarcerated right femoral hernia

15. Postoperative peritoneal adhesions

16. Cholelithiasis with both acute and chronic cholecystitis

17. Ileus due to gallstones which obstruct the intestine

18. Acute obstructive appendicitis

19. Acute gastric ulcer with hemorrhage due to alcohol dependence in remission

20. A patient is admitted with diverticulitis of the large intestine with abscess.

21. Duodenal ulcer with obstruction, perforation, and hemorrhage

22. Bleeding esophageal varices in portal hypertension

Continued

23. The patient is seen by his family physician and diagnosed with gluten-sensitive enteropathy.

24. The patient came to the emergency room with the symptoms of vomiting blood and having very dark stools that appeared to be bloody. The patient is also being treated for congestive heart failure and atrial fibrillation. After study, it was determined the patient had a chronic gastric ulcer with bleeding.

25. A 68-year-old man was admitted to the hospital for bilateral inguinal hernia repair. The patient also had evaluation and treatment of COPD, chronic low back pain, and hypertension while in the hospital. After being prepared for surgery, the patient complained of precordial chest pain. The surgery was cancelled. Cardiac studies failed to find a reason for the chest pain, which resolved later that day.

26. This patient has extensive cellulitis of the abdominal wall due to an infection of the existing gastrostomy site. A feeding tube was inserted four months ago because of the patient's carcinoma of the middle esophagus. The physician confirmed that the responsible organism for the infection is *Staphylococcus aureus*.

27. An elderly man came to Dr. Smith's office complaining of severe epigastric pain. He had experienced some nausea, but no vomiting. Dr. Smith decided to perform studies to rule out cholecystitis and ulcer perforation.

    Impression: Possible cholecystitis or perforated stomach ulcer

28. A 78-year-old woman was admitted to the hospital because of severe rectal bleeding. Because her hemoglobin count was so low, she also received three transfusions of whole blood. A colonoscopy was done, and several ulcers of the rectum were found that later proved to be ulcerative proctitis.

    Discharge diagnoses: Rectal bleeding; acute blood loss anemia; ulcerative proctitis

Diseases of the Skin and Subcutaneous Tissue

OBJECTIVES

After completing this lesson, you should be able to do the following:

- Apply knowledge of current, approved ICD-10-CM coding guidelines to assign and sequence accurate codes for diagnoses related to disorders of the skin and subcutaneous tissue
- Discuss the organism responsible for causing cellulitis and the predisposing conditions for cellulitis
- Identify the major types of skin disorders
- Describe the stages of pressure ulcers

ICD-10-CM

ICD-10-CM Chapter 12, Diseases of skin and subcutaneous tissue, includes categories L00–L99 arranged in the following blocks:

L00–L08	Infections of the skin and subcutaneous tissue
L10–L14	Bullous disorders
L20–L30	Dermatitis and eczema
L40–L45	Papulosquamous disorders
L49–L54	Urticaria and erythema
L55–L59	Radiation-related disorders of the skin and subcutaneous tissue
L60–L75	Disorders of skin appendages
L76	Intraoperative and postprocedural complications of skin and subcutaneous tissue
L80–L99	Other disorders of the skin and subcutaneous tissue

Many codes include laterality, such as L02.522, Furuncle of the left hand and L03.111, Cellulitis of the right axilla. Codes for unspecified sides of the body, such as L02.639, Carbuncle of unspecified foot, also exist.

These conditions normally are treated by dermatologists, internists, and general practitioners.

Cellulitis

Cellulitis is an acute inflammation of a localized area of superficial tissue. Predisposing conditions are open wounds, ulcerations, tinea pedis, and dermatitis, but these conditions need not be present for cellulitis to occur. Physical findings reveal red, hot skin with edema at the site of infection. The area is tender, and the skin surface has a *peau d'orange* (skin of an orange) appearance, with ill-defined borders. Nearby lymph nodes often become inflamed. Cellulitis clears within a few days when treated with antibiotics. In severe cases, abscesses may form that require drainage. However, coders should not assume that mention of redness at the edges of a wound or ulcer represents cellulitis. The normal hyperemia associated with a wound usually extends slightly beyond the wound's edges rather than in the diffuse pattern that characterizes cellulitis. Unless a diagnosis of cellulitis is documented by the physician, a code from category L03 should not be assigned.

The organism responsible for cellulitis is usually *Streptococcus*. There is ordinarily little or no necrosis, suppuration, or abscess, although these occasionally occur when other organisms, such as S*taphylococcus*, are involved. Both abscess and lymphangitis are included in the code for cellulitis of the skin.

Category L03 is further subdivided to identify the site and determine whether the condition is cellulitis or acute lymphangitis.

> **EXAMPLE:** Cellulitis of the left upper arm due to *Streptococcus*:
>
> L03.114 Cellulitis of left upper limb
>
> B95.5 Unspecified Streptococcus as the cause of diseases classified elsewhere

Coding of cellulitis secondary to superficial injury, burn, or frostbite requires two codes: one for the injury and one for the cellulitis. Designation of the principal diagnosis depends on the reason for admission. Cellulitis frequently develops as a complication of chronic skin ulcers (L89, L97, or L98.4). These codes do not include any associated cellulitis, and two codes are required when both conditions are present.

Cellulitis described as gangrenous is classified to code I96, Gangrene, not elsewhere classified rather than to the L03 category. The gangrene is assigned as principal, and the underlying injury or ulcer is assigned as an additional code.

Cellulitis also may be present as a postoperative wound infection or as a result of the penetration of the skin involved in intravenous therapy. It may develop as early as five days postoperatively but often does not appear until a little later.

Dermatitis

Dermatitis is inflammation of the skin. ICD-10-CM classifies dermatitis and eczema to categories L20–L30, depending on the underlying cause and type. Contact dermatitis resulting from substances such as detergents, solvents, oils and greases, drugs and medicines, plants, animal fur, and other chemical products, as well as solar radiation, is reported with a code from categories L23, L24, L25, or L27.

> **EXAMPLE:** Contact dermatitis due to detergents:
>
> L24.0, Irritant contact dermatitis due to detergents

When dermatitis is a reaction to medicine, the coder must first determine whether the condition is a poisoning (incorrect use of a drug) or an adverse effect (due to the proper administration of a drug). A code from categories T36–T50 would be assigned to demonstrate the cause of the dermatitis. The sequencing of the codes will depend on whether the cause is due to a poisoning or to an adverse effect. A poisoning code is always principal, and the dermatitis code would be a secondary code. In the case of an adverse effect, the T36–T50 code would be an additional code.

EXAMPLE: Generalized dermatitis due to penicillin taken correctly as prescribed:

L27.0, Generalized skin eruption due to drugs and medicaments taken internally

T36.0x5A, Adverse effect of penicillin, taken as prescribed

Other examples of codes in these categories include:

- L21.0   Seborrhea capitas (cradle cap)
- L22   Diaper dermatitis
- L23.0   Allergic contact dermatitis due to metals
- L23.2   Allergic contact dermatitis due to cosmetics
- L24.4   Irritant contact dermatitis due to drugs in contact with skin
- L26   Exfoliative dermatitis
- L27.2   Dermatitis due to ingested food
- L28.2   Other prurigo
- L29.3   Anogenital pruritus

Radiation-Related Disorders of the Skin and Subcutaneous Tissue

Category L55 is used to code first, second, and third degree sunburns. Subcategory codes include the following:

- L55.0   Sunburn of first degree
- L55.1   Sunburn of second degree
- L55.2   Sunburn of third degree
- L55.9   Sunburn, unspecified

Also included in this block is radiodermatitis, either acute or chronic. An additional code should be used to identify the source of the radiation.

Disorders of the Appendages

The various category codes included in this block include:

- L60   Nail disorders
- L62   Nail disorders in diseases classified elsewhere
- L63   Alopecia areata
- L64   Androgenic alopecia
- L65   Other nonscarring hair loss
- L66   Cicatricial alopecia (scarring hair loss)
- L67   Hair color and hair shaft abnormalities
- L68   Hypertrichosis
- L70   Acne
- L71   Rosacea
- L72   Follicular cysts of skin and subcutaneous tissue

- L73   Other follicular disorders
- L74   Eccrine sweat disorders
- L75   Apocrine sweat disorders

Categories L63–L68 include many types of disorders of the hair, including alopecia. Codes L63 and L64 describe alopecia areata and androgenic (male-pattern baldness) alopecia. If androgenic alopecia is caused by drug use, an additional code for an adverse effect (T36–T50) should be used to identify the drug. Category L68, Hypertrichosis, is used to describe cases of excess hair, such as Hirsutism, code L68.0.

Various forms of acne are classified to code L70. The subcategory codes include the following:

- L70.0   Acne vulgaris
- L70.1   Acne conglobate
- L70.2   Acne varioliformis
- L70.3   Acne tropica
- L70.4   Infantile acne
- L70.5   Acné excoriée des jeunes filles
- L70.8   Other acne
- L70.9   Acne, unspecified

Ulcers of the Skin

Category L97 is used to report nonpressure chronic ulcer of the lower limb, with additional characters to identify site, laterality, and severity of the ulcers. The severity codes are used to describe breakdown of the skin, fat layer exposed, necrosis of muscle, or necrosis of bone.

Underlying conditions causing the skin ulcers should be reported as well. The underlying condition should be sequenced first. Some underlying causes include atherosclerosis, chronic venous hypertension, diabetic ulcers, postphlebitic syndromes, postthrombotic syndrome, and gangrene.

> **EXAMPLE:**   Chronic ulcer of the left calf due to the patient's diabetes. The fat layer is exposed. Patient is a type 2 diabetic.
>
> Principal diagnosis code is E11.622. Code L97.222 is used as an additional code.

Code L98.4 is used to report nonpressure chronic ulcer of the skin, not elsewhere classified (NEC).

Stasis ulcers are usually due to varicose veins in the lower extremities and are reported with codes from category I83, Varicose veins of the lower extremities, rather than to conditions of the skin.

Pressure (Decubitus) Ulcer

Codes from category L89, Pressure ulcer, are combination codes that identify the site of the pressure ulcer as well as the stage of the ulcer. The ICD-10-CM classifies pressure ulcer stages based on severity, which is designated by stages I–IV, unspecified stage, and unstageable. Assign as many codes from category L89 as needed to identify all the pressure ulcers the patient has, if applicable.

Assignment of the code for unstageable pressure ulcer should be based on the clinical documentation. These codes are used for pressure ulcers whose stage cannot be clinically determined, such as when the ulcer is covered by eschar or has been treated with a skin or muscle graft. Unstageable pressure ulcers are different from pressure ulcers where the stage is not documented. These are coded as unspecified stage.

Assignment of the pressure ulcer stage should be guided by clinical documentation at the stage or documentation of the terms found in the Alphabetic Index. No code is assigned if the documentation states that the pressure ulcer has completely healed. However, pressure ulcers described as healing should be assigned the appropriate pressure ulcer stage based on the documentation in the medical record. If the documentation does not provide information about the stage of the healing pressure ulcer, assign the appropriate code for unspecified stage. Finally, if the patient is admitted with a pressure ulcer at one stage and it progresses to a higher stage, assign the code for the highest stage reported at that site.

For the pressure ulcer stage codes, code assignment may be based on medical record documentation from clinicians who are not the patient's provider (that is, physician or other qualified healthcare practitioner legally accountable for establishing the patient's diagnosis), since this information is typically documented by other clinicians involved in the care of the patient (for example, nurses often document the pressure ulcer stages). However, the diagnosis of pressure ulcer must be documented by the patient's provider. If there is conflicting medical record documentation, either from the same clinician or different clinicians, the patient's attending provider should be queried for clarification.

According to the National Pressure Ulcer Advisory Panel, the descriptions of the four stages are as follows:

Stage I   Intact skin with nonblanching erythema (a reddened area on the skin). This may be referred to as discoloration of the skin without ulceration.

Stage II   Abrasion, blister, shallow open ulcer or crater, or other partial-thickness skin loss.

Stage III Full-thickness skin loss involving damage or necrosis into subcutaneous soft tissues.

Stage IV   Full-thickness skin loss with necrosis of soft tissues through to the muscle, tendons, or tissues around underlying bone

ICD-10-CM Coding Guidelines have very specific guidelines for coding pressure ulcers:

Unstageable pressure ulcers: Assignment of the code for unstageable pressure ulcer should be based on the clinical documentation. These codes are used for pressure ulcers whose stage cannot be clinically determined (for example, the ulcer is covered by eschar or has been treated with a skin or muscle graft) and pressure ulcers that are documented as deep tissue injury but not documented as due to trauma. This code should not be confused with the codes for unspecified stage (L89.—9). When there is no documentation regarding the stage of the pressure ulcer, assign the appropriate code for unspecified stage (L89.—9).

Documented pressure ulcer stage: Assignment of the pressure ulcer stage code should be guided by clinical documentation of the stage or documentation of the terms found in the Alphabetic Index. For clinical terms describing the stage that are not found in the Alphabetic Index, and there is no documentation of the stage, the provider should be queried.

Patients admitted with pressure ulcers documented as healed: No code is assigned if the documentation states that the pressure ulcer is completely healed.

Patients admitted with pressure ulcers documented as healing: Pressure ulcers described as healing should be assigned the appropriate pressure ulcer stage code based on the documentation in the medical record. If the documentation does not provide information about the stage of the healing pressure ulcer, assign the appropriate code for unspecified stage.

If the documentation is unclear as to whether the patient has a current (new) pressure ulcer or if the patient is being treated for a healing pressure ulcer, query the provider.

Patient admitted with pressure ulcer evolving into another stage during the admission: If a patient is admitted with a pressure ulcer at one stage, and it progresses to a higher stage, assign the code for the highest stage reported for that site. (ICD-10-CM Official Coding Guidelines for Coding and Reporting, 2013 found on the Centers for Disease Control and Prevention website).

Pilar Cyst or Trichilemmal Cyst

Pilar cysts are epidermal cysts formed by an outer wall of keratinizing epithelium without a granular layer, similar to the normal epithelium of the hair follicle at and distal to the sebaceous duct. Pilar cysts are common, occurring in five to ten percent of the population. About 90 percent of pilar cysts occur on the scalp and are almost always benign. In two percent of pilar cysts, single or multiple foci of proliferating cells lead to proliferating tumors, often called proliferating trichilemmal cysts. Although typically benign, they may be locally aggressive, becoming large and ulcerated. Pilar cysts are not the same as sebaceous cysts. Codes used to report these conditions are as follows:

L72.1   Pilar and trichilemmal cysts
     L72.11   Pilar cyst
     L72.12   Trichilemmal cyst

Chapter 13: ICD-10-CM Exercises

Review the following statements and cases and assign the appropriate codes:

1. Diaper rash

2. Cellulitis of the foot; culture reveals *Staphylococcal aureus*

3. Infected ingrown toenail

4. Postinfectional skin cicatrix

5. Allergic urticaria

6. Pressure ulcer of sacrum, stage III

7. Erythema multiforme

8. Acute lymphadenitis

9. A 24-year-old female patient is seen by her dermatologist for acne that has persisted since the birth of her baby some eight months ago. While reviewing the patient's medical record, the dermatologist notes that the patient had a history of high blood pressure during her pregnancy along with a history of hyperemesis gravidarum. The physician diagnoses her acne and prescribes medicine. In addition, he takes her blood pressure, which was within the normal range (120/80).

    Impression: Acne

    Code(s):

10. An elderly female patient with the acute onset of erythema, tenderness, and swelling in the right posterior neck area was evaluated in the nursing home. The provisional diagnosis was cellulitis, and IV antibiotic treatment was begun. A CT scan revealed a medium-sized soft-tissue mass in the right posterior neck with the possibility of some abscess formation.

    Diagnoses: Cellulitis; possible abscess formation

11. Actinic keratosis due to tanning bed overuse

12. Nonhealing chronic ulcer of the skin of the right thigh; necrosis of the bone

13. Three-week-old Infant is seen in doctor's office with cradle cap

14. The patient was seen for treatment of a fine rash that had developed on the patient's trunk and upper extremities over the last three to four days. The patient was diagnosed with hypertension seven days ago and started on Ramipril 10 mg daily. The physician determined the rash to be dermatitis due to the Ramipril. The Ramipril was discontinued, and the patient was prescribed a new antihypertensive medication, Captopril. In addition, the physician prescribed a topical cream for the localized dermatitis.

15. Irritant contact dermatitis due to cosmetics; Cystic acne

    The patient was seen with extensive inflammation and irritation of the skin of both upper eyelids and under her eyebrows that was spreading to her temples and forehead. Upon questioning the patient, the physician learned that she had recently used new eye cosmetics. The physician had examined the patient during a prior visit for cystic acne. During this visit, the physician also examined the patient's cystic acne on her forehead and jawline. The patient was advised to continue using the medication previously prescribed. The patient was also advised to immediately discontinue use of any makeup on the face and was given a topical medication to resolve the inflammation, which was an adverse effect of the cosmetics.

16. Cellulitis of the right upper shoulder treated with intravenous antibiotics. The patient is also a known morphine drug abuser and exhibited considerable drug-seeking behavior and continuously requested morphine. All narcotics were discontinued, and the patient exhibited no drug withdrawal symptoms.

17. Gangrenous diabetic skin ulcer of the right mid-foot due to peripheral circulatory disorder

18. The elderly nursing home patient was admitted to the hospital with a severe pressure ulcer on the left buttock, stage I and pressure ulcers on both heels: stage I on the right heel and stage II on the left. Patient has Alzheimer's disease.

19. Severe inflammation in varicose ulcer of the lower left leg

20. Keloid of right hand from previous third degree burns

Diseases of the Musculoskeletal System and Connective Tissue

OBJECTIVES

After completing this lesson, you should be able to do the following:

- Apply knowledge of current, approved ICD-10-CM coding guidelines to assign and sequence accurate codes for diagnoses related to diseases of the musculoskeletal system and connective tissue such as arthritis, systemic lupus erythematosus, and intervertebral disk disorders

- Define pathologic fracture and explain the coding rules relating to a pathologic fracture

ICD-10-CM

ICD-10-CM Chapter 13, Diseases of the musculoskeletal system and connective tissue (M00–M99), organizes the musculoskeletal system and connective tissue in the following blocks:

M00–M02	Infectious arthropathies
M05–M14	Inflammatory polyarthropathies
M15–M19	Osteoarthritis
M20–M25	Other joint disorders
M26–M27	Dentofacial anomalies [including malocclusion] and other disorders of jaw
M30–M36	Systemic connective tissue disorders
M40–M43	Deforming dorsopathies
M45–M49	Spondylopathies
M50–M54	Other dorsopathies
M60–M63	Disorders of muscles
M65–M67	Disorders of synovium and tendon
M70–M79	Other soft tissue disorders
M80–M85	Disorders of bone density and structure

M86–M90	Other osteopathies
M91–M94	Chondropathies
M95	Other acquired disorders of the musculoskeletal system and connective tissue
M96	Intraoperative and postprocedural complications and disorders of musculoskeletal system, not elsewhere classified
M99	Biomechanical lesions, not elsewhere classified

Recurrent bone, joint, or muscle conditions that are the results of a healed injury are also found in Chapter 13.

The musculoskeletal system provides support and movement of body parts. The skeleton is the framework of the body and is composed of bone and cartilage. The bones provide a place for muscles and supporting structures to attach. The muscles allow the movement of the various body parts by means of contraction and relaxation of muscle fibers.

Orthopedics is the branch of medicine that deals with the preservation and restoration of bones and associated structures. An orthopedist or orthopedic surgeon is one who practices orthopedics. Rheumatology is the branch of medicine that deals with rheumatic disorders, which affect the connective tissues of the body, especially the joints and related structures. A rheumatologist is a specialist in rheumatology. Rheumatologists most often treat the various forms of arthritis.

To report musculoskeletal diseases accurately, the following information must be known:

- Anatomic site, such as cervical spine, hip, or ankle

- Severity (acute versus chronic)

- Underlying cause, such as neurogenic, drug-induced, or postsurgical

Site and Laterality

Most of the codes in Chapter 13 include site and laterality designations. The site indicates the bone, joint, or muscle involved. For example, stress fracture of right tibia (M84.361), rheumatoid bursitis of left shoulder (M06.212), and muscle spasm of back (M62.830). For some conditions where more than one bone, joint, or muscle is usually involved, such as osteoarthritis, there is a multiple sites code available. For categories where no multiple site code is provided and more than one bone, joint, or muscle is involved, multiple codes should be used to indicate the different sites involved.

Bone versus Joint

For certain conditions, the bone may be affected at the upper or lower end (for example, avascular necrosis of bone, M87, Osteoporosis, M80, M81). Though the portion of the bone affected may be at the joint, the site designation will be the bone, not the joint (ICD-10-CM Official Guidelines for Coding and Reporting, 2013 found at the Centers for Disease Control and Prevention).

Acute Traumatic versus Chronic or Recurrent Musculoskeletal Conditions

Many musculoskeletal conditions are a result of previous injury or trauma to a site, or are recurrent conditions. Bone, joint or muscle conditions that are the result of a healed injury are usually found in Chapter 13. Recurrent bone, joint or muscle conditions are also usually found in Chapter 13. Any current, acute injury should be coded to the appropriate injury code from Chapter 19. Chronic or recurrent conditions should generally be coded with a code from Chapter 13. If it is difficult to determine from the documentation in the record which code is best to describe a condition, query the provider.

Arthritis and Other Arthropathies

The first block of the chapter on diseases of the musculoskeletal system and connective tissue for infectious arthropathies includes arthropathies due to microbiological agents. To assist coding professionals on the correct usage of categories M00–M02, new guidelines provide definitions for direct and indirect infection.

Distinction is made between the following types of etiological relationships:

- Direct infection of joint—where organisms invade synovial tissue and microbial antigen is present in the joint.

- Indirect infection—which may be of two types: a reactive arthropathy, where microbial infection of the body is established, but neither organisms nor antigens can be identified in the joint, and a postinfective arthropathy, where microbial antigen is present, but recovery of an organism is inconstant, and evidence of local multiplication is lacking.

Arthritis may be a common manifestation of other conditions. In some cases, combination codes are available, and in other cases dual coding is necessary. Some examples include the following:

- M11.812   Arthritis of the left shoulder due to dicalcium phosphate crystals
- C95.90, M35.1   Arthritis due to leukemia
- D66, M36.2   Arthritis due to hemophilia
- A54.42   Gonococcal arthritis
- C90.0-, M35.1   Arthritis in myelomatosis

Infectious Arthritis

Infectious, septic, and bacterial arthritis (M00) is caused when pyogenic bacteria or other infectious agents invade the synovial tissue. The type of organism infecting the joint determines the course of the illness. Adults are most commonly infected with gonococci, staphylococci, streptococci, or pneumococci. Children are frequently infected with staphylococci, *Haemophilus influenzae*, and gram-negative bacilli. Septic arthritis at any age may be caused by viral pathogens (for example, rubella, mumps, or hepatitis B).

Rheumatoid Arthritis

Categories M05–M08, Rheumatoid arthritis (RA) and other inflammatory polyarthropathies, classify a chronic, crippling condition that affects the joints of the hands, feet, wrists, elbows, and ankles. Periods of remission and exacerbation occur in afflicted patients. Although the exact etiology of the disease is unknown, immunologic changes and tissue hypersensitivity, complicated by a cold and damp climate, may have a contributory effect. The synovial membranes are primarily affected. The joints become inflamed, swollen, and painful, as well as stiff and tender. A characteristic sign is the formation of nodules over body surfaces. During an active period, the patient suffers from malaise, fever, and sweating. RA occurs in women two to three times more frequently than in men.

The coder is reminded to also code any manifestations documented, such as enteritis or ulcerative colitis. Juvenile arthritis, unspecified, is assigned to M08. Juvenile arthritis begins before the age of 16 years and has similar characteristics to adult RA. Juvenile RA is clinically divided into various subtypes, such as systemic, pauciarticular, and polyarticular. Systemic onset is sometimes called Still's disease. High fever, rash, splenomegaly, adenopathy, and neutrophilic leukocytosis are characteristics of this subtype. Approximately 40 percent of children with the condition are affected by the pauciarticular subtype, which is characterized by iritis, joint deformity, and unequal leg length. The polyarticular type, which also affects approximately 40 percent of children with the disease, is characterized by symptoms and onset similar to adult RA.

Osteoarthrosis and Allied Disorders

Categories M15–M19, Osteoarthritis, include conditions described as osteoarthrosis, osteoarthritis (OA), degenerative arthritis, and degenerative joint disease (DJD). Osteoarthritis is characterized by erosion of cartilage (either primary or secondary to trauma or other conditions), which becomes soft, frayed, and thinned. This condition is also known as degenerative joint disease and osteoarthrosis. Three-digit codes identify the site of the arthritis. The fourth characters identify whether the arthritis is unilateral or bilateral, and sixth characters identify laterality. Osteoarthritis is reported with codes M15 through M19, with the exception of osteoarthritis of the spine, which is assigned to category M47. Examples of codes in categories M15–M19 include the following:

- M16   Osteoarthritis of hip

     M16.0   Bilateral primary osteoarthritis of hip

     M16.1   Unilateral primary osteoarthritis of hip

         M16.10   Unilateral primary osteoarthritis, unspecified hip

         M16.11   Unilateral primary osteoarthritis, right hip

         M16.12   Unilateral primary osteoarthritis, left hip

     M16.2   Bilateral osteoarthritis resulting from hip dysplasia

     M16.3   Unilateral osteoarthritis resulting from hip dysplasia

         M16.30   Unilateral osteoarthritis resulting from hip dysplasia, unspecified hip

         M16.31   Unilateral osteoarthritis resulting from hip dysplasia, right hip

         M16.32   Unilateral osteoarthritis resulting from hip dysplasia, left hip

     M16.4   Bilateral post-traumatic osteoarthritis of hip

Other Joint Disorders

Categories M20–M25 identify a variety of other joint disorders, including deformity of fingers and other limbs. These category codes include the following:

- M20   Acquired deformity of fingers and toes
- M21   Other acquired deformities of limbs
- M22   Disorders of patella
- M23   Internal derangement of knee
- M24   Other specific joint derangements
- M25   Other joint disorder, not elsewhere classified

Current injuries of the knee and other joints are classified as trauma and found in Chapter 19 in ICD-10-CM. Recurrent dislocations or derangements are assigned to codes M23 and M24. The common conditions included in these code categories include the following:

- M20.1   Hallux valgus (acquired)
- M20.3   Hallux varus (acquired)
- M20.4   Other hammer toe(s) (acquired)
- M21.4   Flat foot [pes planus] (acquired)

- M22.0- Recurrent dislocation of patella
- M23.00 Cystic meniscus, unspecified meniscus
- M23.4- Loose body in knee
- M23.5- Chronic instability of knee
- M24.6- Ankylosis of joint
- M25.0- Hemarthrosis
- M25.4- Effusion of joint
- M25.5- Pain in joint

Laterality plays an important part in the codes in Chapter 13:

- M25.51 Pain in shoulder

  M25.511 Pain in right shoulder

  M25.512 Pain in left shoulder

  M25.519 Pain in unspecified shoulder
- M24.62 Ankylosis, elbow

  M24.621 Ankylosis, right elbow

  M24.622 Ankylosis, left elbow

  M24.629 Ankylosis, unspecified elbow

Systemic Connective Tissue Disorders

Systemic lupus erythematosus (SLE) is a chronic generalized connective tissue disorder ranging from mild to fulminating. It is marked by skin eruptions, arthralgia, fever, leukopenia, visceral lesions, and other constitutional symptoms. ICD-10-CM classifies SLE to code M32. Fourth characters differentiate among drug-induced SLE, SLE with organ or system involvement, and other forms of SLE. Fifth characters under M32.1 identify the specific organ system involved. Examples include the following:

- M32.11 Endocarditis in SLE
- M32.12 Pericarditis in SLE
- M32.13 Lung involvement in SLE
- M32.14 Glomerular disease in SLE
- M32.15 Tubulo-interstitial nephropathy in SLE

Category M33 is used to report the types of dermatopolymyositis, such as juvenile or polymyositis. Codes in M36, Systemic disorders of connective tissue in diseases classified, are always used as additional codes. The coder is instructed to "code first underlying condition." Examples of codes in M36 include the following:

- M36.0 Dermatopolymyositis in neoplastic disease
- M36.1 Arthropathy in neoplastic disease
- M36.2 Hemophilic arthropathy
- M36.3 Arthropathy in other blood disorders

Dorsopathies

Codes describing intervertebral disk disorders and spondylosis, as well as other back disorders, are included in the blocks M40–M54, Dorsopathies. Codes M40–M43 are used for reporting deforming dorsopathies, codes M45–M49 are used to report spondylopathies, and M50-M54 are used to report other dorsopathies.

Some of the common disorders reported with codes in block M40–M43 include kyphosis and lordosis, scoliosis, spinal osteochondrosis, spondylolysis, spondylolisthesis, spinal fusion, and torticollis.

Codes from M45–M49 (Spondylopathies) include such conditions as Ankylosing spondylitis (M45), Infection of intervertebral disc (M46.3), and Spondylosis (M47). Some common conditions reported with category codes M50–M54 include various cervical, thoracic, and lumbosacral disc disorders (with myelopathy or radiculopathy).

Osteomyelitis

Category M86, Osteomyelitis, is further subdivided to fourth-character subcategories that describe acute or chronic osteomyelitis and site. The fifth digit subclassification identifies the laterality of the site involved. An additional code should be assigned that describes the organism involved. Examples of codes in M86 include the following:

- M86.0   Acute hematogenous osteomyelitis

  M86.00   Acute hematogenous osteomyelitis, unspecified site

  M86.01   Acute hematogenous osteomyelitis, shoulder

  M86.011   Acute hematogenous osteomyelitis, right shoulder

  M86.012   Acute hematogenous osteomyelitis, left shoulder

  M86.019   Acute hematogenous osteomyelitis, unspecified shoulder

  M86.02   Acute hematogenous osteomyelitis, humerus

  M86.021   Acute hematogenous osteomyelitis, right humerus

  M86.022   Acute hematogenous osteomyelitis, left humerus

  M86.029   Acute hematogenous osteomyelitis, unspecified humerus

- M86.1   Other acute osteomyelitis
- M86.2   Subacute osteomyelitis
- M86.3   Chronic multifocal osteomyelitis
- M86.4   Chronic osteomyelitis with draining sinus
- M86.5   Other chronic hematogenous osteomyelitis

Coding of Pathological Fractures

Some current musculoskeletal conditions in Chapter 13 are the result of a previous injury or trauma to a site, and others are recurrent conditions. Any acute injury is coded using codes from Chapter 19 in ICD-10-CM. However, some fractures that are included in Chapter 13 are current events. Examples of these are stress fractures (M84.3) and pathological fractures (M84.4 through M84.6). ICD-10-CM has different categories and subcategories for pathologic fractures: category M80, Osteoporosis with current pathological fractures; subcategory M84.4, Pathological fracture, not elsewhere classified; M84.5, Pathological fracture in neoplastic disease; and subcategory M84.6, Pathological fracture in other disease.

When coding pathological or spontaneous fractures using ICD-10-CM, the fifth character identifies the specific site, and the sixth character demonstrates laterality. These fracture codes require an appropriate seventh character to identify the episode of care. For example, the seventh character A indicates initial encounter for the fracture, and the seventh character D is used for subsequent encounters for fracture with routine healing. Examples of subsequent treatment are cast change or removal, removal of external or internal fixation device, medication adjustment, other aftercare, and follow-up visits. The use of these seventh characters for the episode of care is new in ICD-10-CM and is also used for traumatic fractures coded in Chapter 19. Other seventh characters used include G for subsequent encounter for fracture with delayed healing, K for subsequent encounter for fracture with nonunion, and P for subsequent encounter for malunion. Seventh character S is used for encounters for the treatment of sequelae or residuals after the acute phase of the fracture has ended.

Sequencing of codes for pathological fractures is dependent on the reason for admission. If the patient is admitted for treatment of the fracture, the principal diagnosis code would be for the fracture; however, if treatment is directed toward the underlying condition, that condition is sequenced first, with an additional code for the pathological fracture.

A code for both a traumatic fracture and a pathological fracture of the same bone should not be reported.

Osteoporosis

Osteoporosis is a systemic condition, meaning that all bones of the musculoskeletal system are affected. Therefore, site is not a component of the codes under category M81, Osteoporosis without current pathological fracture. The site codes under category M80, Osteoporosis with current pathological fracture, identify the site of the fracture, not the osteoporosis.

Category M80, Osteoporosis with current pathological fracture, is for patients who have a current pathologic fracture at the time of the encounter. The codes under M80 identify the site of the fracture. A code from category M80, not a traumatic fracture code, should be used for any patient with known osteoporosis who suffers a fracture, even if the patient had a minor fall or trauma, if that fall or trauma would not usually break a normal, healthy bone. In category M80, Osteoporosis with current pathological fracture, a fragility fracture is defined as a fracture sustained with trauma no more than a fall from a standing height or less that occurs under circumstances that would not cause a fracture in a normal, healthy bone.

Category M81, Osteoporosis without current pathological fracture, is for use for patients with osteoporosis who do not currently have a pathologic fracture due to osteoporosis, even if they have had a fracture in the past. For patients with a history of osteoporotic fractures, status code Z87.310, Personal history of (healed) osteoporosis fracture, should follow the code from M81.

Stress Fractures

Stress fractures are due to repetitive force and are classified to category M84.3. External cause codes may be used to identify the cause of the fracture: for example, code Y93.01, Walking, marching and hiking. The external cause code would be an additional code and not the principal diagnosis. Fatigue fracture, march fracture, and stress reaction fracture are all terms classified to M84.3 in ICD-10-CM.

Intraoperative and Postprocedural Complications

Intraoperative and postprocedural complications of the musculoskeletal system are included in Chapter 13 in ICD-10-CM. In addition to the codes for hemorrhage, hematoma, and accidental puncture or laceration, there are codes specific to musculoskeletal complications, such as subcategory M96.6, Fracture of bone following insertion of orthopedic implant, joint prosthesis.

Review the following statements and cases and assign the appropriate codes:

1. Displacement of thoracic intervertebral disk

2. Pathologic fracture of the vertebra due to osteoporosis, initial encounter

3. Acquired talipes left

4. Systemic lupus erythematosus

5. Acute osteomyelitis of ankle due to *Staphylococcus*

6. Pathologic fracture of the vertebra due to metastatic carcinoma of the bone from the lung

7. Nonpyogenic arthritis of the hip due to *staphylococcal* infection

8. Charcot's arthritis due to diabetes

9. Acute polymyositis; thoracogenic scoliosis

10. Patient is diagnosed with juvenile rheumatoid arthritis, systemic onset of both knees.

11. Dupuytren's contracture

12. Outpatient visit: The patient sustained a cervical fracture in an automobile accident six years ago. He has been experiencing paresthesia at C3–C4 for two years. The symptoms are worsening with pain in his neck and radiating through his arms.

    Impression: Cervical stenosis

    Code(s):

13. Emergency department visit: An elderly farmer was brought to the emergency department with severe nausea and vomiting. Two days ago, he developed diarrhea and now is slightly dehydrated. The patient has a history of arthritis, for which he is on medication. The patient had a CABG three months ago. Laboratory work revealed: Stool sample with *Giardia lamblia*. The patient was rehydrated and released on antidiarrheal medication. He was given pain medication for his arthritis.

    Impression: Gastroenteritis, *Giardia*; dehydration; arthritis

    Code(s):

14. Inpatient admission: The patient was admitted with known traumatic arthritis and ankylosis of the right hip due to an old fracture of the femoral neck sustained after a fall. Patient history revealed arteriosclerotic cardiovascular disease. The patient underwent hip replacement surgery and was released to rehabilitation services.

    Discharge diagnoses: Arthritis and ankylosis of the right hip secondary to old fracture; arteriosclerotic cardiovascular disease

    Code(s):

15. Chief complaint: Sore right knee

    History of present illness: Patient notes that he was moving some boxes over the weekend. He notes that on 1/28, his right knee became sore and swollen. On 1/30, he had shaking, fevers, and chills. He now presents for evaluation. When seen in the office, he denied a history of coughing or other illness. There was no history of trauma to the knee.

    The patient's right knee is swollen, which has limited his ability to move. There is no medial or lateral joint line discomfort and no pain on palpation of the patella. Negative apprehension sign for subluxation. The medial and lateral collateral ligaments are stable. Stress testing of the cruciates was not performed due to the effusion and the lack of reliability of testing with large effusion. There were no tender femoral groin nodes. After suitable prep, while in the office, aspiration was performed on the right knee. Approximately 80 cc of a purulent, turbid-appearing fluid was aspirated. Laboratory work was done. The cultures showed *S. aureus* with oxacillin sensitivity (*methicillin-susceptible Staphylococcal aureus*, or MSSA). The patient was informed of the results and the need for admission to the hospital.

    Hospital course: The patient was admitted on 1/31 after three days of pain in the knee followed by shaking and chills. Aspiration in the office indicated the patient had purulent, turbid-appearing fluid. On admission, he was started on IV antibiotics and was seen in consultation by an infectious disease practitioner. The consultant's impression was that the patient had septic arthritis. He was taken to surgery on 2/1, at which time he underwent arthroscopic irrigation and debridement with tube placement. He was maintained on drip-suck irrigation. He was taken back to surgery on 2/4 for repeat irrigation and debridement. Postoperatively, his temperature resolved. The organism was also sensitive to Timentin. He was then discharged on intravenous Timentin. He had instructions to return to the office for follow-up.

    Discharge diagnosis: Septic arthritis due to *Staph aureus*, MSSA

    Code(s):

16. This 86-year-old male patient was diagnosed with left upper lobe lung carcinoma, approximately 10 years ago. He is now seen now for a fracture of the shaft of the right femur. After work-up, the patient was diagnosed with metastatic bone cancer (from the lung), resulting in the fracture. The work-up did not reveal any recurrence of the primary site.

17. Patient with senile osteoporosis is seen for the complaints of severe back pain with no history of trauma. X-rays revealed pathological compression fractures of several lumbar vertebrae.

18. Aneurysmal bone cyst of the left tibia

19. Traumatic arthritis of the right ankle, due to chronic dislocation of the ankle

20. Acute and chronic gouty arthritis

21. Pyogenic (bacterial) arthritis of the hip

22. Chronic bucket-handle tear of the lateral meniscus of the right knee

23. Low back pain

Continued

24. The patient is a 75-year-old male with complaints of low back pain radiating down his left leg down to the foot. The pain has become progressively worse over the last four months. MRI of the lumbar scan showed degenerative disc disease at L2-3 and L3-4; past medical history includes hypertension and CAD.

25. A 86-year-old woman complains of severe joint pain in the hips and knees. Work-up revealed rheumatoid arthritis with myopathy.

26. The patient was seen in the emergency department with complaints of severe neck pain that radiated into both his arms, with numbness and shock-like pains down his body. The MRI showed spinal stenosis at C3-4 and C5-6.

27. The patient was seen in the emergency department with severe chest pain and coughing. Work-up for MI showed no evidence of heart disease. The patient admitted to recovering from pneumonia six weeks ago, and the physician diagnosed the chest pain as costochondritis secondary to coughing from the pneumonia.

28. Patient was seen for a subsequent visit for a healing pathological fracture of the right femur. Patient has metastatic carcinoma of the bone from breast cancer five years ago.

29. Lyme disease with associated arthritis

30. Recurrent dislocation of left shoulder

31. Patient is seen in the emergency department with degenerative arthritis of the hips, knees, and spine. The elderly patient is in a significant degree of pain. The patient also suffers from hypertension and has CAD. Patient had a quadruple bypass 10 years ago with reocclusion of the arteries and is complaining of angina.

32. The 14-year-old female was diagnosed four years ago with scoliosis secondary to neurofibromatosis, type 2, and did well with a brace for all this time. Patient also suffers from mild, persistent asthma, which is currently under good control. The patient is in good health and admitted for surgical fusion of the T1-L4 vertebrae and insertion of an interbody fusion device.

33. Juvenile rheumatoid arthritis, occurring only in both ankles

Diseases of the Genitourinary System

OBJECTIVES

After completing this lesson, you should be able to do the following:

- Apply knowledge of current, approved ICD-10-CM coding guidelines to assign and sequence accurate codes related to diseases of the genitourinary system
- Discuss the major disorders of the genitourinary system
- Identify documentation in the health record that may signify renal failure
- Understand the major gynecologic disorders

ICD-10-CM

These conditions are most often treated by urologists, gynecologists, and general surgeons.
Chapter 14 of ICD-10-CM includes categories N00–N99 arranged in the following blocks:

N00–N08	Glomerular diseases
N10–N16	Renal tubulo-interstitial diseases
N17–N19	Acute kidney failure and chronic kidney disease
N20–N23	Urolithiasis
N25–N29	Other disorders of kidney and ureter
N30–N39	Other diseases of the urinary system
N40–N53	Diseases of male genital organs
N60–N65	Disorders of breast
N70–N77	Inflammatory diseases of female pelvic organs
N80–N98	Noninflammatory disorders of female genital tract
N99	Intraoperative and postprocedural complications and disorders of genitourinary system, not elsewhere classified

Chronic Kidney Disease

Chronic kidney disease (CKD) is usually the result of a gradually progressive loss of renal function. Its causes include chronic glomerular diseases, chronic infections, congenital anomalies, vascular diseases, obstructive processes, collagen diseases, nephrotic agents, and endocrine diseases.

CKD produces major changes in all body systems, resulting in a multitude of complications, including anemia, cardiomyopathy, brittle fingernails, pulmonary edema, increased susceptibility to respiratory infections, metabolic acidosis, and fluid overload. Hemodialysis or peritoneal dialysis can help control some of the manifestations of end-stage renal disease (ESRD).

ICD-10-CM classifies CKD to category N18. Fourth character subcategory codes identify the stage and severity of the disease:

- N18.1   Chronic kidney disease, stage I
- N18.2   Chronic kidney disease, stage II (mild)
- N18.3   Chronic kidney disease, stage III (moderate)
- N18.4   Chronic kidney disease, stage IV (severe)
- N18.5   Chronic kidney disease, stage V
- N18.6   End-stage renal disease
- N18.9   Chronic kidney disease, unspecified

The stage is based on the patient's glomerular filtration rate, which is a test that measures how well the kidneys are working. It is a measurement of how much liquid waste is passing from the blood into the urine each minute and how much creatinine is being eliminated. Normal values are between 90 ml/min and 110 ml/min.

If both a stage of CKD and ESRD are documented, assign code N18.6 only. When N18.6 is used, the coder is instructed to use an additional code to identify dialysis status (Z99.2).

Additional codes should be reported to identify any associated manifestations and kidney transplant status. Patients who have undergone a kidney transplant may still have some type of chronic kidney disease, as the kidney transplant may not have fully restored all kidney function. Code Z94.0, Kidney transplant status, can be assigned, along with the appropriate CKD code for those patients who have had a kidney transplant. The "Use additional code to identify kidney transplant status" under category code N18 provides this instruction.

Use of a N18 code with Z94.0 does not necessarily indicate transplant rejection or failure. Patients with mild or moderate CKD following a transplant should not be coded as having transplant failure, unless it is documented in the medical record. For patients with severe CKD or ESRD, it is appropriate to assign code T86.1—Complications of transplanted organ, kidney transplant—when kidney transplant failure is documented. If CKD is present after kidney transplant, and it is unclear from the documentation whether there is transplant failure or rejection, it is necessary to query the provider.

Documentation that may signify renal failure in the health record includes the following:

- Significantly elevated values of serum creatinine or blood urea nitrogen (BUN), or diminished creatinine clearance
- Specific clinical and laboratory findings such as anemia, hyperphosphatemia, hypocalcemia, hyperkalemia, acidemia, renal osteodystrophy, and uremic symptoms, including nausea, vomiting, itching, hemorrhagic conditions, hypertension, edema, dyspnea, lethargy, and coma

However, the coder needs more than an abnormal laboratory finding to add an additional diagnosis. Remember to always query the physician regarding the specific diagnosis being treated when it is not clearly documented.

Acute Kidney Disease

Acute kidney disease and disorders and acute tubular-interstitial diseases are assigned to category N17, with the fourth character subcategories identifying the presence of tubular necrosis, acute cortical necrosis, or medullary necrosis. Acute renal failure typically develops over a short period of time as part of another illness and is generally reversible and is corrected as the underlying disease is treated or controlled. Acute kidney failure or acute kidney injury, nontraumatic, is reported with N17.9. A traumatic kidney injury is reported with S37.0.

Nephrotic Syndrome

Nephrotic syndrome is characterized by proteinuria, hypoalbuminemia, hyperlipidemia, and edema. It is not a disease itself but, rather, results from a specific glomerular disease that indicates renal damage. ICD-10-CM classifies nephrotic syndrome to category N04, which further subdivides to identify the specific type of lesion involved, such as diffuse membranous glomerulonephritis, minor glomerular abnormality, or diffuse mesangial proliferative glomerulonephritis.

Other ICD-10-CM categories from the block glomerular diseases (N00–N08) are used to report:

- N00   Acute nephritic syndrome
- N01   Rapidly progressive nephritic syndrome
- N02   Recurrent and persistent hematuria
- N03   Chronic nephrotic syndrome
- N05   Unspecified nephritic syndrome
- N06   Isolated proteinuria with specified morphological lesion
- N07   Hereditary nephropathy, NEC
- N08   Glomerular disorders in diseases classified elsewhere

When reporting N08, the coder is advised to code the underlying disease first.

Pyelonephritis

Pyelonephritis, also known as pyelitis, is a pus-forming infection of the kidney. Tubulo-interstitial nephritis, including acute pyelonephritis (N10), is usually caused by an infection that moves upward from the lower urinary tract into the kidneys. Its symptoms include fever, chills, pain, nausea, and the frequent need to urinate. Urinalysis will reveal many bacteria and white blood cells, and antibiotic therapy is prescribed. Chronic tubulo-interstitial nephritis, including pyelonephritis (N11.9), develops after a bacterial kidney infection. Most cases are linked to some form of blockage, such as a stone in the ureter. Treatment includes removal of the blockage and long-term use of antibiotics. Code N16, Renal tubulo-interstitial disorders in diseases classified elsewhere, is reported when the pyelonephritis occurs secondary to another disease, such as tuberculosis. The underlying disease should be coded and sequenced first. For example, pyelitis in leukemia is coded N16, with the diagnosis code from categories C81–C85 or C96 sequenced first.

Cystitis

Cystitis is inflammation of the urinary bladder. Symptoms include dysuria, suprapubic pain, lower back pain, hematuria, and the need and desire to urinate often. It may be caused by bacterial infection, a stone, or a tumor. Most common in women, this condition is often recurrent. Most cases are due to a vaginal infection that extends through the urethra to the bladder. Cystitis in men is due to urethral or prostatic infections or catheterizations. Depending on the diagnosis, treatment may include antibiotics, drinking more liquids, bed rest, drugs to control bladder spasms, and surgery, when needed.

ICD-10-CM classifies cystitis to category N30, with the fourth character describing the specific type and the fifth character identifying the presence or absence of hematuria. An instruction at the beginning of this category advises that an additional code from Chapter 1 of the ICD-10-CM code book, Infectious and parasitic diseases, should be assigned to identify the organism involved. Examples from category N30 include the following:

- N30.0   Acute cystitis

    N30.00   Acute cystitis without hematuria
    N30.01   Acute cystitis with hematuria
- N30.1   Interstitial cystitis (chronic)
- N30.2   Other chronic cystitis
- N30.3   Trigonitis
- N30.4   Irradiation cystitis
- N30.8   Other cystitis
- N30.9   Cystitis, unspecified

The fifth characters under codes N30.1–N30.9 also differentiate between with and without hematuria.

Without further specification, cystitis is reported with code N30.9.

An additional code should be assigned when the underlying organism is identified. The coder should not arbitrarily add an additional diagnosis on the basis of an abnormal laboratory finding alone. The physician should always be queried when the specific diagnosis is not clearly stated in the health record.

> **EXAMPLE:**   Urinary tract infection due to Shiga toxin-producing *E. coli*: O157
> N30.00, Urinary tract infection
> B96.21, Shiga toxin-producing Escherichia coli O157

Calculus of Urinary Tract

Calculi of the urinary tract can occur in the kidney, ureter, urethra, or bladder. The renal pelvis or calyces of the kidneys are a common place of formation. Calculi can vary in size and may be solitary or multiple. They may remain in the renal pelvis or enter into the ureter. In some instances, calculi can cause obstruction, which may result in hydronephrosis. Calculi are classified to several different codes in ICD-10-CM, depending on the location of the calculus, as follows:

- N20.0   Calculus of kidney
- N20.1   Calculus of ureter
- N20.2   Calculus of kidney with calculus of ureter
- N20.9   Urinary calculus, unspecified
- N21.0   Calculus in bladder
- N21.1   Calculus in urethra
- N21.8   Other lower urinary tract calculus
- N21.9   Calculus of lower urinary tract, unspecified

Vesicoureteral Reflux

Vesicoureteral reflux is a backflow of urine from the bladder into the ureters. It is characterized by abdominal or flank pain, persistent or recurrent urinary infection, dysuria (pain with voiding), and frequency or urgency of urination. Moreover, pyuria, hematuria, proteinuria, or bacteriuria may accompany vesicoureteral reflux. ICD-10-CM classifies vesicoureteral reflux to subcategory N13.7. Fifth and sixth characters add specificity:

- N13.70   Vesicoureteral-reflux, unspecified
- N13.71   Vesicoureteral-reflux without reflux nephropathy
- N13.72   Vesicoureteral-reflux with reflux nephropathy
  - N13.721   Vesicoureteral-reflux with reflux nephropathy without hydroureter, unilateral
  - N13.722   Vesicoureteral-reflux with reflux nephropathy without hydroureter, bilateral
  - N13.729   Vesicoureteral-reflux with reflux nephropathy without hydroureter, unspecified

Examples of other codes from category, N13, Obstructive and reflux uropathy, include the following:

- N13.1   Hydronephrosis with ureteral stricture, not elsewhere classified
- N13.2   Hydronephrosis with renal and ureteral calculous obstruction
- N13.3   Other and unspecified hydronephrosis
- N13.4   Hydroureter
- N13.5   Crossing vessel and stricture of ureter without hydronephrosis
- N13.6   Pyonephrosis
- N13.7   Vesicoureteral-reflux
- N13.8   Other obstructive and reflux uropathy
- N13.9   Obstructive and reflux uropathy, unspecified

Urethral or Ureteral Stricture

Urethral stricture is an abnormal narrowing of the urethra due to inflammation, scarring, or pressure from outside the body. ICD-10-CM classifies urethral stricture to category N35, which further subdivides to identify the underlying cause, such as infection or postoperative development. When the urethral stricture is specified as congenital, code Q64.39, Other atresia and stenosis of urethra and bladder neck should be assigned. Stricture of the ureter is reported with N13.5, Crossing vessel and structure of ureter without hydronephrosis.

Other Urinary Symptoms

Other urinary symptoms include hematuria, urinary retention, urinary dysuria, and urinary incontinence.

Hematuria

Hematuria, code R31, or blood in the urine, can produce a red-to-brown discoloration, depending on the amount of blood in the urine and the acidity of the urine. Microscopic hematuria may cause no discoloration and would be detected only by chemical testing or a microscopic examination. This condition may present with pain or may be painless. ICD-10-CM classifies hematuria, unspecified, to subcategory R31.9. Fourth characters in R31 identify gross, R31.0 (visually seen by the eye), and microscopic hematuria. Microscopic hematuria is reported with either R31.1, Benign essential microscopic hematuria, or R31.2, Other microscopic hematuria.

Urinary Retention

Urinary retention is a buildup of urine in the bladder. Its causes may be related to loss of muscle tone in the bladder, nerve damage, a blocked urethra, or use of a narcotic painkiller, such as morphine. ICD-10-CM classifies urinary retention to category R33, Retention of urine, which is located in the chapter for symptoms, signs, and abnormal clinical and laboratory findings. The category further subdivides to identify specific types of urine retention, including the following:

- R33.0   Drug induced retention of urine
- R33.8   Other retention of urine
- R33.9   Retention of urine, unspecified

Urinary Dysuria

Urinary dysuria is painful urination. This condition may suggest an inflammation or irritation of the urethra or bladder neck. ICD-10-CM classifies this condition to code R30, Pain associated with micturition. Subcategory codes include the following:

- R30.0   Dysuria
- R30.1   Vesical tenesmus
- R30.9   Painful micturition, unspecified

Urinary Incontinence

Urinary incontinence is a loss of urine without warning and may be associated with many conditions. ICD-10-CM classifies many types of urinary incontinence to subcategory N39.4, which further subdivides to type, such as urge or stress incontinence, continuous leakage, and nocturnal enuresis. Examples of codes used to specify urinary incontinence include the following:

- N39.41   Urge incontinence
- N39.42   Incontinence without sensory awareness
- N39.43   Post-void dribbling
- N39.44   Nocturnal enuresis
- N39.45   Continuous leakage
- N39.46   Mixed incontinence

Other symptoms related to the genitourinary system include urinary frequency (R35.0), nocturia (R35.1), polyuria (R35.8), and anuria and oliguria (R34).

Cystostomy Complications

Code N99.51 is used to report various complications of a cystostomy. These include hemorrhage, infection, and malfunction. N99.518 is used to report other cystostomy complication.

Z Codes of Interest

Admission as an inpatient may be necessary for fitting or adjustment of a dialysis catheter or for adequacy testing for dialysis. The following codes are used to identify admissions for these situations:

- Z49.01   Encounter for fitting and adjustment of extracorporeal dialysis catheter
- Z49.02   Encounter for fitting and adjustment of peritoneal dialysis catheter

- Z49.31   Encounter for adequacy testing for hemodialysis
- Z49.32   Encounter for adequacy testing for peritoneal dialysis

If a patient is admitted for other medical reasons but receives dialysis while in the facility, code Z99.2, Dependence on renal dialysis, is used as an additional code. The reason for admission would be the principal diagnosis. There may be instances when the physician documents that the patient is noncompliant with renal dialysis; code Z91.15, Patient's noncompliance with renal dialysis, would be assigned.

Disorders of the Prostate

Disorders of the prostate are common problems experienced by men and often treated on an outpatient basis. Two of the most common problems are enlarged prostate and prostatitis.

Enlarged Prostate

ICD-10-CM uses the term *enlarged prostate* rather than *hypertrophy* or *hyperplasia*. Enlarged prostate commonly occurs in men older than 60 years. The prostate gland, which encircles the urethra at the base of the bladder, becomes enlarged and presses on the urethra, obstructing the flow of urine from the bladder. Symptoms of benign prostatic hyperplasia (BPH) include urinary frequency, urgency, nocturia, incontinence, and hesitancy, decreased size and force of stream, and/or complete urinary retention. Straining to void may rupture veins of the prostate, causing hematuria.

A diagnosis of BPH is made by a rectal examination that finds the prostate enlarged and with a rubbery texture. Urinalysis shows white blood cell count, red blood cell count, albumin, bacteria, and blood. Cystoscopy reveals the extent of enlargement. A post-voiding cystogram shows the amount of residual urine in the bladder.

Enlarged prostate is coded to N40. A "use additional code" under code N40.1 and N40.3 reminds the coder to code the associated symptoms, if any, when coding an enlarged prostate. Some of the associated symptoms include incomplete bladder emptying (R39.14), straining on urination (R39.16), urinary obstruction (N13.8), nocturia (R35.1), and urinary urgency (R39.15).

The fourth characters include the following:

- N40.0   Enlarged prostate without lower urinary tract symptoms
- N40.1   Enlarged prostate with lower urinary tract symptoms
- N40.2   Nodular prostate without lower urinary tract symptoms
- N40.3   Nodular prostate with lower urinary tract symptoms

Benign and malignant neoplasms of the prostate are excluded from this category.

Prostatitis

Prostatitis is inflammation of the prostate that may present in an acute form (N41.0) or a chronic form (N41.1). Additional codes may be assigned to identify the underlying organism, such as *Staphylococcus aureus*.

Mild and moderate prostatic intraepithelial neoplasia (PIN I and PIN II) should be coded to N42.3. An excludes note directs the coder to use code D07.5 when severe prostatic dysplasia (PIN III) is diagnosed.

Hydrocele

A hydrocele is an accumulation of fluid in any saclike cavity or duct, specifically in the membrane surrounding the testicles or along the spermatic cord. ICD-10-CM classifies hydroceles to category N43, which includes hydrocele involving the spermatic cord, testis, or tunica vaginalis. This category further subdivides to identify specific types, such as encysted or infected. When the hydrocele is described as congenital, the correct code assignment is P83.5, Congenital hydrocele.

Breast Disorders

Disorders of the breast that are not neoplastic in nature are classified to categories N60–N65. The codes within this block include the following:

- N60 Benign mammary dysplasia
- N61 Inflammatory disorders of the breast
- N62 Hypertrophy of the breast
- N63 Unspecified lump of the breast
- N64 Other disorders of breast
- N65 Deformity and disproportion of reconstructed breast

Some of the more commonly used codes include the following:

- N60.0   Cyst of the breast
- N60.2   Fibroadenosis of breast
- N60.3   Fibrosclerosis of breast
- N62   Hypertrophy of breast
- N64.1   Fat necrosis of breast
- N64.2   Atrophy of breast
- N64.53 Retraction of nipple
- N64.81 Ptosis of breast

Reconstruction after breast surgery is reported with code Z42.1, Encounter for breast reconstruction following mastectomy. When a mammoplasty is done to reduce breast size, code N62, Hypertrophy of the breast, is used. When mammoplasty is done to increase breast size, code Z41.1, Encounter for cosmetic surgery, is used.

Gynecologic Disorders

Gynecologic disorders include endometriosis, cervicitis, genital prolapse, cervical dysplasia, ovarian cysts, and ovarian dysfunction.

Endometriosis

Endometriosis is the presence of endometrial tissue outside the lining of the uterine cavity. It is generally confined to the pelvic area but can appear anywhere in the body. The classic symptom of endometriosis is dysmenorrhea, which can cause constant pain in the lower abdomen, vagina, posterior pelvis, and back. ICD-10-CM classifies endometriosis to category N80, which further subdivides to identify the specific sites affected:

- N80.0 Endometriosis of the uterus
- N80.1 Endometriosis of the ovary
- N80.2 Endometriosis of the fallopian tube
- N80.3 Endometriosis of the pelvic peritoneum

Cervicitis

Cervicitis (N72) is a sudden or long-term inflammation of the cervix, which is the lower, narrow end of the uterus. In the acute phase, swelling, redness, and bleeding occur. This condition also can produce a foul-smelling discharge, pelvic pain, itching, and/or a burning of the outer genital area. Chronic cervicitis, a persistent inflammation of the cervix, produces symptoms similar to the acute type.

When the specific organism causing the cervicitis is documented, codes from Chapter 1 in ICD-10-CM are used. For example: Chlamydia cervicitis (A56.09), Gonococcal cervicitis (A54.03), and Herpesviral cervicitis (A60.03).

Genital Prolapse

Genital prolapse is the falling, sliding, or sinking of the uterus or vagina from its normal position or place. ICD-10-CM classifies female genital prolapse to category N81, which further subdivides to identify the extent of the disease and associated conditions, such as cystocele, cystourethrocele, rectocele, urethrocele, and proctocele. The major subcategory codes include the following:

- N81.0   Urethrocele
- N81.1   Cystocele
- N81.2   Incomplete uterovaginal prolapse
- N81.3   Complete uterovaginal prolapse
- N81.4   Uterovaginal prolapse, unspecified
- N81.5   Vaginal enterocele
- N81.6   Rectocele
- N81.8   Other female genital prolapse
- N81.9   Female genital prolapse, unspecified

Dysplasia of Female Organs

Cervical intraepithelial neoplasia (CIN), or cervical dysplasia, is the condition of abnormal cell structure in the cervical epithelium. It can be a premalignant condition of abnormal growth of squamous cells on the surface of the cervix. This condition is classified to code N87.0 for CIN I or mild cervical dysplasia, and code N87.1 for CIN II or moderate cervical dysplasia. Dysplasia classified as CIN III is considered carcinoma *in situ* of the service and is reported with code D06.-.

ICD-10-CM codes N90.0 and N90.1 are used to report vulvar intraepithelial neoplasia (VIN) I and II, respectively. If the condition is described as carcinoma *in situ* of the vulva, severe dysplasia of the vulva, or vulvar intraepithelial neoplasia (VIN III), ICD-10-CM code D07.1 is used to classify the disease.

Vaginal intraepithelial neoplasia (VAIN) is a premalignant condition involving the vagina. It is classified as VAIN I, II, and III. As with CIN and VIN, VAIN III is considered carcinoma *in situ*. VAIN III is reported with D07.2. A pathological examination is necessary to code these conditions correctly.

Ovarian Cysts

Ovarian cysts may be nonneoplastic or neoplastic in origin. Nonneoplastic cysts include follicular, lutein, corpus luteum, and endometrial or chocolate cysts. These conditions are reported with category N83, Noninflammatory disorders of ovary, fallopian tube, and broad ligament. Subcategory codes include the following:

- N83.0   Follicular cyst of the ovary
- N83.1   Corpus luteum cyst
- N83.2   Other and unspecified ovarian cyst

Chapter 15: ICD-10-CM Exercises

Review the following statements and cases and assign the appropriate codes:

1. Chronic kidney disease, stage III

2. Acute pyelonephritis due to Shiga toxin-producing *E. coli*, unspecified

3. Staghorn calculus of kidney

4. Hematuria, frequency of urination, and nocturia

5. Fibroadenosis of right breast

6. Mild cervical dysplasia

7. Vesicoureteral reflux with bilateral reflux nephropathy

8. Absence of menstruation

9. Postmenopausal bleeding

10. Diabetic nephrotic syndrome, type I

11. Female infertility secondary to Stein-Leventhal syndrome

12. Acquired multiple cysts of the left kidney

13. A 77-year-old woman was admitted to the hospital with intense pain described as renal or ureteral colic. An intravenous pyelogram (IVP) revealed a relatively large stone in the left kidney with some renal dysfunction and another stone in the distal ureter on the left side. During the IVP, the patient began to complain of some chest pain, and a cardiology consultation was requested.

    Discharge diagnoses: Left ureteral calculus; left renal calculus; chest pain

14. A 27-year-old woman complaining of elevated temperature was seen in the emergency department by her family physician; high temperature was 102°F. She also complained of lower back pain and frequent urination. A urinalysis was done, and a bacterial organism (*Pseudomonas*) was identified. She was given a prescription for antibiotics and released.

    Discharge diagnosis: Severe, acute cystitis

15. A 36-year-old woman was admitted to the hospital with complaints of severe and constant pain in the lower abdomen and back. Upon questioning by the physician, the patient stated that her menstrual periods were very painful, often causing her to have to miss work. A diagnostic workup revealed endometriosis that involved the fallopian tubes, both ovaries, and the uterus. A hysterectomy and bilateral salpingo-oophorectomy were done, and the patient was later discharged from the hospital in good condition.

    Discharge diagnosis: Endometriosis of the fallopian tubes, both ovaries, and uterus

16. Donation of kidney to a family member with ESRD

17. Congenital polycystic kidney disease

18. Status post right nephrectomy

19. Patient has hydronephrosis with chronic pyelitis; pyelonephritis, chronic, due to *E. coli*.

20. A young man is diagnosed with an abscess of the left testis due to group B *Streptococcus*.

21. Chronic cystitis with hematuria due to *Pseudomonas*.

22. A young woman was diagnosed with infertility due to congenital anomaly of the fallopian tube.

23. Hypertensive heart and kidney disease with stage V chronic kidney disease and congestive heart failure

24. Female patient has postcatheterization stricture of the urethra with resulting urinary incontinence.

25. The patient is seen for a scheduled renal dialysis session for ESRD.

26. Patient is seen by her plastic surgeon, because she is concerned about her previously implanted breast prostheses. She has had no problems but wishes to have the implants removed.

27. Urethral stricture secondary to gonorrheal infection

28. This male patient complained of lower abdominal pain and the inability to urinate over the past 24 hours. After study, the patient was diagnosed as having acute kidney failure due to acute tubular necrosis, caused by a urinary obstruction. The urinary obstruction was a result of the patient's benign prostatic hypertrophy. The patient was treated with medications and the acute kidney failure was resolved prior to discharge.

29. Patient is currently being treated for chronic kidney disease, stage 3. She has previously undergone a kidney transplant but still continues to suffer from chronic kidney disease. This patient is also treated for hypothyroidism following removal of the thyroid for thyroid carcinoma. At this time, there is no longer evidence of an existing thyroid malignancy.

30. A patient complaining of fever, malaise, and right flank pain has a urinalysis performed that showed bacteria of more than 100,000/ml present in the urine, and subsequent urine culture shows *Proteus* growth as the cause of the urinary tract infection. The patient was treated with intravenous antibiotics. The patient also has a history of repeated UTIs over the past several years. The final diagnosis is urinary tract infection due to *Proteus*.

Pregnancy, Childbirth, and the Puerperium

OBJECTIVES

After completing this lesson, you should be able to do the following:

- Apply knowledge of current, approved ICD-10-CM guidelines to assign and sequence accurate codes for diagnoses related to complications of pregnancy, childbirth, and the puerperium
- Apply knowledge of ICD-10-CM coding guidelines to assign and sequence accurate codes for the different types of abortions and the possible complications of each
- List the criteria for assignment of code O80, Normal delivery
- Discuss the Z codes that are appropriate to abortion, pregnancy, childbirth, and the postpartum period
- Discuss the use of seventh characters in relation to pregnancy coding in ICD-10-CM

ICD-10-CM

Chapter 15 of the ICD-10-CM code book classifies conditions that affect the management of pregnancy, childbirth, and the puerperium (or postpartum period). Many conditions that are classified to other chapters in the code book are reclassified to Chapter 15 when they occur during pregnancy, childbirth, or in the postpartum period. Any condition occurring during these periods is considered a complication, unless the physician specifically states that it is unrelated to the pregnancy. When a physician states that the pregnancy is unrelated to the condition being treated, the condition is coded and Z33.1—Pregnant state, incidental—is assigned as an additional code.

Chapter 15, Pregnancy, childbirth, and the puerperium of ICD-10-CM includes categories O00–O9A arranged in the following blocks:

O00–O08	Pregnancy with abortive outcome
O09	Supervision of high-risk pregnancy
O10–O16	Edema, proteinuria, and hypertensive disorders in pregnancy, childbirth, and the puerperium

O20–O29	Other maternal disorders predominantly related to pregnancy
O30–O48	Maternal care related to the fetus and amniotic cavity and possible delivery problems
O60–O77	Complications of labor and delivery
O80, O82	Encounter for delivery
O85–O92	Complications predominantly related to the puerperium
O94–O9A	Other obstetric conditions, not elsewhere classified

The conditions described in these categories are most often treated by obstetricians and gynecologists.

Ectopic and Molar Pregnancy

Ectopic and molar pregnancies as well as other abnormal products of conception are classified to categories O00–O01 as follows:

- O00 Ectopic pregnancy
- O01 Hydatidiform mole
- O02 Other abnormal product of conception

An ectopic pregnancy is a pregnancy that arises from implantation of the ovum in other than the uterine cavity. Almost all ectopic pregnancies are tubal (occurring in the fallopian tube). Other sites include the peritoneum, ovary, or cervix. Subcategory codes include the following:

- O00.0 Abdominal pregnancy
- O00.1 Tubal pregnancy
- O00.2 Ovarian pregnancy
- O00.8 Other ectopic pregnancy
- O00.9 Ectopic pregnancy, unspecified

A molar pregnancy is an abnormal pregnancy in which a nonviable fertilized egg implants in the uterus but fails to develop. It may or may not contain any fetal tissue. It is characterized by the presence of a hydatid mole or hydatidiform mole. Hydatid moles are classified to category O01, and fourth characters indicate whether it is a classical or complete hydatidiform mole, an incomplete or partial hydatidiform mole, or unspecified. Code O01.0, for example, is a classical (complete) hydatidiform mole. Other types of abnormal products of conception include blighted ovum and nonhydatidiform mole. These conditions are reported with O02.0.

Abortion

The word *abortion* in the disease classification of ICD-10-CM refers to the expulsion or extraction from the uterus of all or part of the products of conception (with or without an identifiable embryo or a nonviable fetus weighing less than 500 g). When fetal weight cannot be determined, an estimated gestation of less than 20 completed weeks is considered an abortion. Abortions and the complications that follow abortions, ectopic pregnancies, and molar pregnancies are classified as follows:

- O03 Spontaneous abortion
- O04 Complications following (induced) termination of pregnancy
- O07 Failed attempted termination of pregnancy

Codes in subcategories O03.0– O03.4 indicate that the abortion is incomplete, meaning there are retained products of conception. Codes in subcategories O03.5–O03.9 indicate that the abortion is complete. If no documentation is found indicating incomplete or complete spontaneous abortion, the code for complete is used. Category O04 is used for complications of induced termination of pregnancy. ICD-10-CM does not contain codes for illegally induced abortions or unspecified abortions.

The fourth characters for O03 and O04 indicate the presence or absence of a complication arising during the same admission or encounter as that of the abortion:

- O03.0   Genital tract and pelvic infection following incomplete spontaneous abortion
- O03.1   Delayed or excessive hemorrhage following incomplete spontaneous abortion
- O03.2   Embolism following incomplete spontaneous abortion
- O03.3   Other and unspecified complications following incomplete spontaneous abortion

  O03.31   Shock following incomplete spontaneous abortion
  O03.32   Renal failure following incomplete spontaneous abortion
  O03.33   Metabolic disorder following incomplete spontaneous abortion

- O04.5   Genital tract and pelvic infection following (induced) termination of pregnancy
- O04.6   Delayed or excessive hemorrhage following (induced) termination of pregnancy

An additional code from Z3A would be used to indicate, if known, the weeks of gestation.

The elective abortion (without complication) code has been moved to code Z33.2, Encounter for elective termination of pregnancy, in Chapter 21 of ICD-10-CM.

Examples

- A patient is admitted following an incomplete spontaneous abortion with delayed and excessive hemorrhage. Code O03.1, Delayed or excessive hemorrhage following incomplete spontaneous abortion, is assigned along with a code from category Z3A.

- A patient is readmitted to the facility following an elective termination of pregnancy. She is diagnosed with a pelvic infection. Code O04.5, Genital tract and pelvic infections following (induced) termination of pregnancy, is assigned in this situation. A code from Z3A is also assigned.

One week following a spontaneous abortion, the patient is readmitted and diagnosed with oliguria. The documentation suggests that the etiology is retained fetal tissue. Code O03.82 is assigned, even though the abortion took place on an earlier encounter. A code from Z3A is assigned as an additional code.

Missed Abortion

A missed abortion (O02.1) is an early fetal death before completion of 20 weeks gestation, with retention in the uterus. A loss of the fetus after 20 weeks gestation is considered a missed intrauterine fetal death (O36.4-).

Coders frequently confuse the clinical condition of missed abortion with spontaneous abortion. A missed abortion is the retention in the uterus of a fetus that has died. The death is indicated by cessation of growth, hardening of the uterus, loss of size of the uterus, and absence of fetal heart tones after they have been heard on previous examinations. In contrast to a spontaneous abortion, no products of conception, fetal parts, or tissue are expelled from the uterus when the patient has a missed abortion. All of the uterine contents remain in the uterus. When a spontaneous abortion occurs, the woman experiences one or more of the classic symptoms, such as uterine contractions, uterine hemorrhage, dilation of the cervix, and presentation or expulsion of all or part of the products of conception.

Abortion Resulting in Live Fetus

Code O60.1-, Preterm labor with preterm delivery, should be assigned for an attempted abortion resulting in a liveborn infant. In addition to code O60.1-, a code to describe the outcome of delivery (Z37) is assigned. A code from category Z3A for the weeks of gestation will also be assigned. A code for the procedure performed for the termination of pregnancy also should be assigned.

> **EXAMPLE:** Attempted therapeutic abortion resulting in liveborn fetus:
>
> O60.10X0, Preterm labor with preterm delivery, unspecified trimester
>
> Z37.0, Outcome of delivery, single liveborn
>
> Z3A.00, unspecified weeks of gestation

Complications Specific to Multiple Gestation

In rare instances, a patient who is pregnant with multiple fetuses is admitted for a spontaneous abortion for one or more of the fetuses. However, one or more live fetuses remain in utero. In these instances, no code from category O00–O08 is assigned; rather, assign a code from subcategory O31.1-, Continuing pregnancy after spontaneous abortion of one fetus or more is assigned.

Death of one fetus or more after 20 weeks gestation would be reported with a code from O31.2:

O31.2   Continuing pregnancy after intrauterine death of one fetus or more
    O31.20   Continuing pregnancy after intrauterine death of one fetus or more, unspecified trimester
    O31.21   Continuing pregnancy after intrauterine death of one fetus or more, first trimester
    O31.22   Continuing pregnancy after intrauterine death of one fetus or more, second trimester
    O31.23   Continuing pregnancy after intrauterine death of one fetus or more, third trimester

Recurrent Pregnancy Loss

A recurrent pregnancy loss is the spontaneous expulsion of a dead or nonviable fetus in three or more consecutive pregnancies at about the same period of development. If the patient with recurrent pregnancy loss is admitted for a spontaneous abortion, use appropriate code from category O03. For a patient who is not pregnant and is diagnosed as having recurrent pregnancy loss, code O26.2-. Code O09.29-, Supervision of pregnancy with other poor reproductive or obstetric history, is used to describe supervision of a high-risk pregnancy in a patient with a history of recurrent pregnancy loss but without a diagnosis of recurrent pregnancy loss.

Pregnancy

Codes from Chapter 15 are used only on maternal records and never on newborn infant records.

Two common definitions that should be reviewed are for the peripartum and postpartum periods. The peripartum period is defined as the last month of pregnancy to five months postpartum. The postpartum period begins immediately after delivery and continues for six weeks following delivery. Normal pregnancies are intrauterine. Following is a guide for determining preterm, term, and prolonged postterm pregnancies:

- Preterm describes delivery before 37 completed weeks of gestation
- Term describes delivery between 38 and 40 weeks of gestation
- Postterm describes delivery between 40 and 42 completed weeks of gestation
- Prolonged describes delivery after 42 completed weeks of gestation

In the Alphabetic Index, long listings of conditions appear under Pregnancy, Labor, Delivery, and Puerperium. Indentations often are used under these main terms, so extreme care should be taken in locating and selecting the appropriate code.

Trimester

The majority of the codes in Chapter 15 have a character that indicates the trimester of the pregnancy in which the admission or encounter occurred. Trimesters are counted from the first day of the last menstrual period. They are defined as follows:

- First trimester—less than 14 weeks, 0 days
- Second trimester—14 weeks, 0 days, to less than 28 weeks, 0 days
- Third trimester—28 weeks, 0 days, until delivery

However, the assignment of the trimester must be based on the documentation of the provider. The provider may refer to the weeks of gestation instead of specifically stating the trimester. On rare occasions, a hospitalization may encompass more than one trimester. When this occurs, the trimester character for the condition is based on when the complication occurred rather than simply on discharge. For example, a patient may be admitted at the end of the first trimester with preeclampsia and remains hospitalized into the second trimester. The code would reflect a complication occurring in the first trimester.

Not every code in Chapter 15 includes a trimester component. This generally happens when a condition occurs only in a specific trimester or the specific condition is such that a trimester is not necessary.

Each category that includes codes for trimester has a code for unspecified trimester. The unspecified trimester code should rarely be used, such as when the documentation in the record is insufficient to determine the trimester, and it is not possible to obtain clarification.

Weeks of Gestation

Codes from category Z3A are used on the maternal record to indicate the weeks of gestation of the pregnancy for all pregnancies. It would be used as an additional code after any codes for complications of pregnancy, childbirth, and the puerperium:

- Z3A.0   Weeks of gestation of pregnancy, unspecified or less than 10 weeks

  Z3A.00   Weeks of gestation of pregnancy not specified

  Z3A.01   Less than 8 weeks of pregnancy not specified

  Z3A.08   8 weeks gestation of pregnancy

  Z3A.09   9 weeks gestation of pregnancy

- Z3A.4   Weeks of gestation of pregnancy, weeks 40 or greater

  Z3A.40   40 weeks gestation of pregnancy

  Z3A.41   41 weeks gestation of pregnancy

  Z3A.42   42 weeks gestation of pregnancy

  Z3A.49   Greater than 42 weeks gestation of pregnancy

Normal Delivery

Category O80, Encounter for full-term uncomplicated delivery, is assigned when all the following criteria are met:

- Delivery of a full-term, single, healthy, liveborn infant
- Delivery without prenatal or postpartum complications classifiable to Chapter 15
- Cephalic or occipital presentation with spontaneous, vaginal delivery requiring minimal or no assistance, with or without episiotomy, without fetal manipulation (for example, rotation, version) or instrumentation (forceps)
- Any antepartum complication that the patient may have had during the pregnancy must be resolved before delivery

Code O80 is always the principal diagnosis.

Outcome of Delivery

The outcome of delivery, as indicated by a code from category Z37, should be included on all maternal delivery records. This is always an additional, not principal, diagnosis code used to reflect the number and status of babies delivered. Category code Z37 is referenced in the Alphabetic Index under Outcome of delivery.

> **EXAMPLE:** Normal delivery and pregnancy, 40 weeks gestation, single liveborn:
> O80, Normal delivery
> Z3A.40, 40 week gestation of pregnancy
> Z37.0, Outcome of delivery, single liveborn

Fetal Seventh Characters

Many of the codes in Chapter 15 of ICD-10-CM require the use of a seventh character to identify the fetus to which certain complication codes apply:

0—not applicable or unspecified
1—fetus 1
2—fetus 2
3—fetus 3
4—fetus 4
5—fetus 5
9—other fetus

These seventh characters are used for multiple gestations to identify the fetus to which the code applies. The character 0 is used in cases of single gestations or when the documentation does not indicate to which fetus the problem applies. When characters 1 through 9 are used, the expectation is that a code from the multiple gestation category would be used.

The following subcategories or codes require a seventh character extension to identify the fetus for which the complication code applies:

- O31.00–O31.8x9   Complications specific to multiple gestation
- O32.0–O32.9   Maternal care for malpresentation of fetus
- O33.3   Maternal care for disproportion due to outlet contraction of pelvis

- O33.4   Maternal care for disproportion of mixed maternal and fetal origin
- O33.5   Maternal care for disproportion due to unusually large fetus
- O33.6   Maternal care for disproportion due to hydrocephalic fetus
- O35.0–O35.9   Maternal care for known or suspected fetal abnormality and damage
- O36.011–O36.93   Maternal care for other fetal problems
- O40.1–O40.9   Polyhydramnios
- O41.00–O41.93   Other disorders of amniotic fluid and membranes
- O60.10–O60.14   Preterm labor with preterm delivery
- O60.20–O60.23   Term delivery with preterm labor
- O64.0–O64.9   Obstructed labor due to malposition and malpresentation of fetus
- O69.0–O69.9   Labor and delivery complicated by umbilical cord complications

Routine Prenatal Visits

Category Z34 is used for a routine encounter for supervision of a normal pregnancy. It is not used with any other codes in Chapter 15. The fourth characters indicate supervision of a normal first pregnancy (Z34.0), supervision of other normal pregnancy (Z34.8), and supervision of normal pregnancy, unspecified (Z34.9). Fifth characters are used to indicate the trimester during which the encounter occurs.

Prenatal Supervision for High-Risk Pregnancy

If the prenatal outpatient visit is to manage a high-risk pregnancy, a code from Chapter 15 category O09, Supervision of high-risk pregnancy, is used as the first-listed code. The high-risk pregnancy supervision codes are in the obstetric code chapter and not reported with Z codes, as are routine visits. Subcategory codes within category O09 are as follows:

- O09.0   Supervision of pregnancy with history of infertility
- O09.1   Supervision of pregnancy with history of ectopic or molar pregnancy
- O09.2   Supervision of pregnancy with other poor reproductive or obstetric history
- O09.3   Supervision of pregnancy with insufficient prenatal care
- O09.4   Supervision of pregnancy with grand multiparity
- O09.5   Supervision of elderly primigravida and multigravida
- O09.6   Supervision of young primigravida and multigravida
- O09.7   Supervision of high-risk pregnancy due to social problems
- O09.8   Supervision of other high-risk pregnancies
- O09.9   Supervision of high-risk pregnancy, unspecified

Fifth characters add greater specificity and sixth characters identify the trimester during which the encounter is occurring.

An elderly primigravida or multigravida is defined as a woman pregnant at 35 and older at the expected date of delivery. A young primigravida or multigravida is defined as a female less than 16 years old at the expected date of delivery. The coder relies on the physician's documentation to assign these codes—not on the age of the patient alone.

Fetal Complications Affecting the Management of the Pregnancy

Codes from categories O35 and O36 are assigned only when the fetal condition is actually responsible for modifying the management of the mother; that is, by requiring diagnostic studies, additional observation, special care, or termination of the pregnancy. The fact that a fetal condition merely exists does not justify assigning a code from these two categories to the mother's health record. Category codes O35 and O36 have seventh characters, which indicate the fetus that is responsible for the condition.

Subcategory codes from O35 include the following:

- O35.0 Maternal care for (suspected) central nervous system malformation in fetus
- O35.1 Maternal care for (suspected) chromosomal abnormality in fetus
- O35.2 Maternal care for (suspected) hereditary care disease in fetus
- O35.3 Maternal care for (suspected) damage to fetus from viral disease in mother
- O35.4 Maternal care for (suspected) damage to fetus alcohol
- O35.5 Maternal care for (suspected) damage to fetus from drugs
- O35.6 Maternal care for (suspected) damage to fetus by radiation
- O35.7 Maternal care for (suspected) damage to fetus by other medical procedure
- O35.8 Maternal care for other (suspected) fetal abnormality and damage
- O35.9 Maternal care for (suspected) fetal abnormality and damage, unspecified

When in utero surgery is performed, a code from category O35.7- is used on the mother's chart. Examples of procedures include amniocentesis, biopsy, hematological investigation, intrauterine contraceptive device, or other intrauterine surgery. Code O09.82, Supervision of pregnancy with history of in utero procedure during previous pregnancy, is used to report visits during a subsequent pregnancy.

Examples of subcategory codes from O36 include the following:

- O36.0 Maternal care for rhesus isoimmunization
- O36.1 Maternal care for other isoimmunization
- O36.2 Maternal care for hydrops fetalis
- O36.4 Maternal care for intrauterine death
- O36.5 Maternal care for known or suspected poor fetal growth
- O36.6 Maternal care for excessive fetal growth
- O36.7 Maternal care for viable fetus in abdominal pregnancy

Code O36.80 is used for an encounter to determine fetal viability. Code O36.81- is used for an encounter for decreased fetal movement. Examples of codes used include the following:

- O36.80 Pregnancy with inconclusive fetal viability
- O36.81 Decreased fetal movements

    O36.812 Decreased fetal movements, second trimester
    O36.813 Decreased fetal movements, third trimester
    O36.819 Decreased fetal movements, unspecified trimester

Multiple Gestation

Category O30, Multiple gestation, is used to identify twin, triplet, quadruplet, or other specified gestation. Fifth characters under category O30 indicate the number of placentas and amniotic sacs in the pregnancy. Sixth characters indicate the trimester. The coder is instructed to "code also any complications specific to multiple gestation." Examples of codes from O30 include the following:

- O30.0   Twin pregnancy
    - O30.00   Twin pregnancy, unspecified number of placenta and unspecified number of amniotic sacs
    - O30.01   Twin pregnancy, monochorionic/monoamniotic
    - O30.02   Conjoined twin pregnancy
    - O30.03   Twin pregnancy, monochorionic/diamniotic
        - O30.031   Twin pregnancy, monochorionic/diamniotic, first trimester
        - O30.032   Twin pregnancy, monochorionic/diamniotic, second trimester
        - O30.033   Twin pregnancy, monochorionic/diamniotic, third trimester

Also included in O30 is the code for conjoined twin pregnancy, code O30.02, with the sixth characters indicating the trimester.

Other Indications for Care Primarily in Antepartum Period

Many pre-existing conditions, such as diabetes, hypertension, or anemia, may affect or complicate the pregnancy or its management. Moreover, pregnancy may aggravate the pre-existing condition. For this reason, when the pregnancy aggravates the condition or the condition aggravates the pregnancy, the pre-existing or other nonobstetrical condition is reclassified to Chapter 15 of the ICD-10-CM code book. In some cases, the code in the obstetrical chapter completely describes the complication, while in other cases additional codes are required.

Codes from block O10–O16 are used to report pre-existing hypertension, which is always considered a complication of pregnancy. Category codes in this section include the following:

- O10   Pre-existing hypertension complicating pregnancy, childbirth, and the puerperium
- O11   Pre-existing hypertension with pre-eclampsia
- O12   Gestational edema and proteinuria without hypertension
- O13   Gestational hypertension without significant proteinuria
- O14   Pre-eclampsia
- O15   Eclampsia
- O16   Unspecified maternal hypertension

Many women develop transient or gestational hypertension during pregnancy. This condition usually clears when the pregnancy is over. Gestational hypertension is coded to O13, Gestational [pregnancy-induced] hypertension without significant proteinuria. However, when the obstetric patient is experiencing gestational edema or gestational proteinuria, Code O12 is assigned.

When eclampsia occurs, code O15 is used, regardless of whether the hypertension is pre-existing. Eclampsia is the most severe phase of pre-eclampsia, and if left unchecked can result in coma and death.

Categories O20–O28 include codes describing conditions and complications mainly related to pregnancy. The category codes included in this block are as follows:

- O20   Hemorrhage in early pregnancy
- O21   Excessive vomiting in pregnancy
- O22   Venous complications and hemorrhoids in pregnancy
- O23   Infections of genitourinary tract in pregnancy
- O24   Diabetes mellitus in pregnancy, childbirth, and the puerperium
- O25   Malnutrition in pregnancy, childbirth, and the puerperium
- O26   Maternal care for other conditions predominantly related to pregnancy
- O28   Maternal findings on antenatal screening of mother
- O29   Complications of anesthesia during pregnancy

Category O21, Excessive vomiting in early pregnancy, further subdivides to indicate at what point during the pregnancy the vomiting began and the presence or absence of metabolic disturbances. Code O21.0, Mild hyperemesis gravidarum, is reported when vomiting starts before the end of week 20 of gestation. Code O21.1, Hyperemesis gravidarum with metabolic disturbance, is reported when the vomiting starts before the end of the 22nd week with the presence of dehydration, electrolyte imbalance, or carbohydrate depletion. Code O21.2, Late vomiting of pregnancy, is reported when the vomiting begins after the 22nd week of gestation. Code O21.9, Unspecified vomiting of pregnancy, is reported for vomiting as a reason for care when the documentation in the health record does not indicate the length of gestation.

For the most part, these categories require the assignment of an additional code to further specify the condition. For example, subcategory O23.0-, Infections of kidney in pregnancy, requires the assignment of an additional code to specify the type of renal disease.

> **EXAMPLE:**   Term pregnancy, 40 weeks, with chronic kidney infection, delivered:
>
> O23.03, Infection of kidney in pregnancy, third trimester
>
> N15.9, Kidney infection
>
> Z3A.40, 40 weeks gestation of pregnancy
>
> Z37.0, Outcome of delivery code

> **EXAMPLE:**   Pregnancy at 25 weeks gestation with acute cystitis:
>
> O23.12, Infections of bladder in pregnancy, second trimester
>
> N30.00, Acute cystitis
>
> Z3A.25, 25 weeks gestation of pregnancy

> **EXAMPLE:**   Intrauterine pregnancy, 18 weeks gestation with chronic gonorrhea:
>
> O98.212, Gonorrhea complicating pregnancy, second trimester
>
> A54.1-, Gonococcal infection of lower genitourinary tract, unspecified
>
> Z3A.18, 18 weeks gestation of pregnancy

> **EXAMPLE:**   Intrauterine pregnancy, 20 weeks, active cocaine dependence:
>
> O99.322, Drug use complicating pregnancy, second trimester
>
> F14.20, Cocaine dependence
>
> Z3A.20, 20 weeks gestation of pregnancy

Category O24—Diabetes mellitus (DM) in pregnancy, childbirth, and the puerperium—uses fourth characters to indicate whether the diabetes is pre-existing or gestational. Subcategory codes O24.0–O24.3 are used to report complications due to pre-existing diabetes mellitus. These codes identify Type 1 DM, Type 2 DM, and unspecified DM. Fifth characters reflect complications during pregnancy, childbirth, and the puerperium, and sixth characters reflect the trimester. Code O24.4 is used to report gestational diabetes, with sixth characters indicating whether the gestational diabetes is diet-controlled or insulin-controlled. Code Z79.4, Long-term (current) use of insulin, would also be assigned if the pre-existing diabetes mellitus is being treated with insulin. It is not used with the gestational diabetes codes nor with the codes under O24 that indicated insulin-controlled. Code Z86.32, Personal history of gestational diabetes, would be reported on a patient that had gestational diabetes on a previous pregnancy.

Category O29 is used to report complications of anesthesia during pregnancy, such as pulmonary complications, cardiac complications, central nervous system complications, toxic reaction, headache, and other complications.

Preterm Labor and Delivery

Category O60, Preterm labor, is used to report labor with onset of labor before 37 completed weeks of gestation. False labor (O47.0-) and threatened labor (O047.0-) are excluded from this category.

Subcategory code O60.0 is used to report preterm labor without delivery. Fifth characters identify the trimester (second or third) in which the preterm labor began. Subcategory code O60.1 is used to report preterm labor with preterm delivery. The fifth characters indicate both when the labor began and when the delivery occurred:

- O60.12   Preterm labor second trimester with preterm delivery second trimester
- O60.13   Preterm labor second trimester with preterm delivery third trimester
- O60.14   Preterm labor third trimester with preterm delivery third trimester

A seventh character is assigned to each of these codes. Subcategory code O60.2 is used for a term delivery with preterm labor.

Postterm Labor and Delivery

Category O48, Late pregnancy, is used to demonstrate that a woman has passed 40 completed weeks of gestation. Code O48.0, Postterm pregnancy, is used from 40 completed weeks through 42 completed weeks. Code O48.1 is used for pregnancy that has advanced beyond 42 completed weeks.

Alcohol and Tobacco Use during Pregnancy, Childbirth, and the Puerperium

Codes under subcategory O99.31—Alcohol use complicating pregnancy, childbirth, and the puerperium—should be assigned for any pregnancy case when a mother uses alcohol during the pregnancy or postpartum period. A secondary code from category F10, Alcohol related disorders, should also be assigned to identify manifestations of the alcohol use.

Codes under subcategory O99.33—Smoking (tobacco) complicating pregnancy, childbirth, and the puerperium—should be assigned for any pregnancy case when a mother uses any type of tobacco product during the pregnancy or postpartum period. A secondary code from category F17,

Nicotine dependence, or code Z72.0, Tobacco use, should also be assigned to identify the type of nicotine dependence. Some examples of codes include the following:

- O99.31   Alcohol use complicating pregnancy, childbirth, and the puerperium

    O99.310   Alcohol use complicating pregnancy, unspecified trimester

    O99.311   Alcohol use complicating pregnancy, first trimester
    O99.312   Alcohol use complicating pregnancy, second trimester

    O99.313   Alcohol use complicating pregnancy, third trimester

    O99.314   Alcohol use complicating childbirth

    O99.315   Alcohol use complicating the puerperium

- O99.32   Drug use complicating pregnancy, childbirth, and the puerperium
- O99.33   Smoking (tobacco) complicating pregnancy, childbirth, and the puerperium
- O99.34   Other mental disorders complicating pregnancy, childbirth, and the puerperium
- O99.35   Diseases of the nervous system complicating pregnancy, childbirth, and the puerperium

Complications Occurring Mainly in the Course of Labor and Delivery

Complications that can occur in the course of labor and delivery include obstructed labor and trauma to the perineum and vulva.

Category code O63   is used to report long labor. The fourth digit codes represent the stage of the prolonged labor:

- O63.0   Prolonged first stage of labor
- O63.1   Prolonged second stage of labor
- O63.2   Delayed delivery of second twin, triplet, etc.
- O63.9   Long labor, unspecified

Category code O69 is used to report labor and delivery that is complicated by umbilical cord complications. Some examples of codes include the following:

- O69.0   Labor and delivery complicated by prolapse of cord
- O69.1   Labor and delivery complicated by cord around neck, with compression
- O69.2   Labor and delivery complicated by other cord entanglement, with compression
- O69.3   Labor and delivery complicated by short cord
- O69.4   Labor and delivery complicated by vasa previa
- O69.5   Labor and delivery complicated by vascular lesion of the cord—cord bruising, cord hematoma, or thrombosis of umbilical vessels
- O69.8   Labor and delivery complicated by other cord complications

    O69.81   Labor and delivery complicated by cord around neck, without compression

    O69.82   Labor and delivery complicated by cord entanglement, without compression

Code categories O64, O65, and O66 are provided to identify obstructed labor. The ICD-10-CM codes for obstructed labor incorporate the reason for the obstruction into the code; therefore, only one code is required.

The codes for obstructed labor describe various types of obstructed labor, such as obstruction caused by malposition of fetus, obstruction caused by bony pelvis, obstruction caused by abnormal pelvic soft tissues, and locked twins.

The category and subcategory codes include the following:

- O64   Obstructed labor due to malposition and malpresentation of fetus

    O64.0   Obstructed labor due to incomplete rotation of fetal head

    O64.1   Obstructed labor due to breech presentation

    O64.2   Obstructed labor due to face presentation

    O64.5   Obstructed labor due to compound presentation

    O64.8   Obstructed labor due to other malposition and malpresentation

    O64.9   Obstructed labor due to malposition and malpresentation, unspecified

- O65   Obstructed labor due to maternal pelvic abnormality

    O65.0   Obstructed labor due to deformed pelvis

    O65.1   Obstructed labor due to generally contracted pelvis

    O65.2   Obstructed labor due to pelvic inlet contraction

    O65.3   Obstructed labor due to pelvic outlet and mid-cavity contraction

    O65.4   Obstructed labor due to fetopelvic disproportion

    O65.5   Obstructed labor due to abnormality of maternal pelvic organs

    O65.8   Obstructed labor due to other maternal pelvic abnormalities

    O65.9   Obstructed labor due to maternal pelvic abnormality, unspecified

- O66   Other obstructed labor

    O66.0   Obstructed labor due to shoulder dystocia

    O66.1   Obstructed labor due to locked twins

    O66.2   Obstructed labor due to unusually large fetus

    O66.3   Obstruction due to other abnormalities of fetus

    O66.4   Failed trial of labor

    O66.5   Attempted application of vacuum extractor and forceps

    O66.6   Obstructed labor due to other multiple fetuses

    O66.8   Other specified obstructed labor

    O66.9   Obstructed labor, unspecified

Seventh characters identify the fetus involved.

Category O70, Perineal laceration during delivery, is used to identify trauma to the perineum during delivery. The following subcategories identify laceration degrees:

- Subcategory O70.0, First-degree perineal laceration, includes lacerations, ruptures, or tears involving the fourchette, hymen, labia, skin, vagina, or vulva

- Subcategory O70.1, Second-degree perineal laceration, includes lacerations, ruptures, or tears (following episiotomy) that involve the pelvic floor, perineal muscles, or vaginal muscles

- Subcategory O70.2, Third-degree perineal laceration, includes lacerations, ruptures, or tears (following episiotomy) that involve the anal sphincter, rectovaginal septum, or sphincter, not otherwise specified

- Subcategory O70.3, Fourth-degree perineal laceration, includes lacerations, ruptures, or tears of sites classifiable to subcategory O70.1 and also involving the anal mucosa or the rectal mucosa
- Subcategory O70.4, Anal sphincter tear complicating delivery, not associated with third degree perineal laceration
- Subcategory O70.9, Perineal laceration during delivery, unspecified

Category O72, Postpartum hemorrhage, includes fourth character subcategories that identify third stage hemorrhage (retained placenta), immediate postpartum hemorrhage, and delayed and secondary postpartum hemorrhage.

Category O75—Other complications of labor and delivery, not elsewhere classified—includes the following fourth character subcategories:

- O75.0   Maternal distress during labor and delivery
- O75.1   Shock during or following labor and delivery
- O75.2   Pyrexia during labor, not elsewhere classified
- O75.3   Other infection during labor
- O75.4   Other complication of obstetric surgery and procedures
- O75.5   Delayed delivery after artificial rupture of membranes
- O75.8   Other specified complications of labor and delivery
- O75.9   Complication of labor and delivery, unspecified

Complications of the Puerperium

Category O85, Puerperal sepsis, is used to report postpartum sepsis, puerperal peritonitis, and puerperal pyemia. The coder is reminded to use an additional code to identify the infectious agent and to identify severe sepsis, if applicable. Code O86, Other puerperal infections, includes codes for infection of obstetric surgical wound, genital tract infection, pyrexia of unknown origin, and urinary tract infection. Approximately 2–4 percent of women experience a postpartal infection. Code O89 is used to report complications of anesthesia during the puerperium. Code O91 is used when infections of the breast result from pregnancy, the puerperium, and lactation. Examples of codes from O91 include the following:

- O91.0   Infection of nipple associated with pregnancy, the puerperium, and lactation

  O91.01   Infection of nipple associated with pregnancy

  O91.011   Infection of nipple associated with pregnancy, first trimester

  O91.012   Infection of nipple associated with pregnancy, second trimester

  O91.013   Infection of nipple associated with pregnancy, third trimester

  O91.019   Infection of nipple associated with pregnancy, unspecified trimester

  O91.02   Infection of nipple associated with the puerperium

  O91.03   Infection of nipple associated with lactation

- O91.1   Abscess of breast associated with pregnancy, the puerperium, and lactation
- O91.2   Nonpurulent mastitis associated with pregnancy, the puerperium, and lactation

HIV Infection

According to the ICD-10-CM coding guidelines.

> During pregnancy, childbirth or the puerperium, a patient admitted because of an HIV-related illness should receive a principal diagnosis from subcategory O98.7-, Human immunodeficiency [HIV] disease complicating pregnancy, childbirth and the puerperium, followed by the code for the HIV-related illness(es). Patients with asymptomatic HIV infection status admitted during pregnancy, childbirth or the puerperium should receive codes of O98.7- and Z21, Asymptomatic human immunodeficiency virus (HIV) infection status (ICD-10-CM Official Guidelines for Coding and Reporting 2013).

Sequelae of Complications of Pregnancy, Childbirth, and the Puerperium

Code O94, Sequelae of complication of pregnancy, childbirth, and the puerperium, is assigned when a complication evolves into a sequela that continues to require care or treatment after the postpartal period is complete. This code can be used at any time after the postpartum period. As with all late effects, the code for the residual condition is sequenced first, and code O94 is assigned as an additional code.

> **EXAMPLE:** A patient is admitted with postpartum perineum prolapse secondary to a third degree laceration sustained during a delivery nine months ago.
>
> N81.89 Other female genital prolapse
>
> O94 Sequelae of complication of pregnancy, childbirth, and the puerperium

Abuse in a Pregnant Patient

For suspected or confirmed cases of abuse of a pregnant patient, code(s) from subcategories O9A.3, Physical abuse complicating pregnancy, childbirth, and the puerperium; O9A.4, Sexual abuse complicating pregnancy, childbirth, and the puerperium; and O9A.5, Psychological abuse complicating pregnancy, childbirth, and the puerperium, should be sequenced first, followed by the appropriate codes (if applicable) to identify any associated current injury due to physical abuse, sexual abuse, and the perpetrator of abuse.

Sequencing of Codes

For routine outpatient prenatal visits when no complications are present, a code from category Z34, Encounter for supervision of normal pregnancy, should be used as the first-listed diagnosis. These codes should not be used in conjunction with any other Chapter 15 codes.

For routine prenatal visits for patients with high-risk pregnancies, a code from category O09, Supervision of high-risk pregnancy, should be used as the first-listed diagnosis. Secondary Chapter 15 codes may be used in conjunction with these codes if appropriate.

In episodes when no delivery occurs, the principal diagnosis should correspond to the principal complication of the pregnancy which necessitated the encounter. When a delivery occurs, the principal diagnosis should correspond to the main circumstances or complication of the delivery. In cases of cesarean delivery, the selection of the principal diagnosis should be the condition established after study that was responsible for the patient's admission. If the patient was admitted with a condition that resulted in the performance of a cesarean procedure, that condition should be selected as the principal diagnosis. If the reason for the admission or encounter was unrelated to the condition resulting in the cesarean delivery, the condition related to the reason for the admission or encounter should be selected as the principal diagnosis.

Z Codes

Category Z30, Encounter for contraceptive management, is reported for encounters related to the purpose of contraceptive management. Some of the circumstances reported with this include oral contraceptive measures (Z30.02), insertion of intrauterine contraceptive device (Z30.430), sterilization procedures (Z30.2), and surveillance of injectable contraceptive (Z30.42).

Code Z30.2 may be the principal diagnosis or a secondary diagnosis, depending on the circumstances of admission. When the primary purpose of an admission or encounter is for contraceptive management (sterilization), code Z30.2 will be the principal diagnosis, with additional codes reported for concomitant conditions. When sterilization occurs during an obstetric delivery, code Z30.2 will be an additional diagnosis.

Several other categories of Z codes are pertinent to pregnancy, childbirth, and the puerperium. Some Z codes of interest include the following:

- Z41   Genetic carrier
- Z15   Genetic susceptibility to disease
- Z30   Encounter for contraceptive management
- Z31   Encounter for procreative management
- Z32   Encounter for pregnancy test and childbirth and childcare instruction
- Z33   Pregnant state
- Z34   Encounter for supervision of normal pregnancy
- Z36   Encounter for antenatal screening of mother
- Z3A   Weeks of gestation
- Z37   Outcome of delivery
- Z39   Encounter for maternal postpartum care and examination
- Z85.4 Personal history of malignant neoplasm of genital organs

Chapter 16: ICD-10-CM Exercises

Review the following statements and cases and assign the appropriate codes:

1. Hyperemesis gravidarum with dehydration, 12 weeks gestation

2. Uterine pregnancy at 20 weeks gestation with gestational hypertension

3. Failure of lactation

4. 25-week pregnancy with internal hemorrhoids

5. Routine prenatal care, eight weeks gestation, primigravida with no complications

6. Routine postpartum care, no complications

7. Elderly multigravida, 12 weeks, prenatal care, no complications

8. Triplet pregnancy, delivered spontaneously at term, 40 weeks; all liveborn; number of placenta and amniotic sacs not specified

9. Moderate pre-eclampsia complicating pregnancy, 29 weeks gestation

10. Threatened abortion with hemorrhage at 15 weeks gestation

11. Testing of female for genetic disease carrier status

12. Postpartum deep thrombophlebitis; developed two weeks following delivery

13. Incomplete early spontaneous abortion at 16 weeks

14. Missed abortion, 19 weeks gestation

15. Induced abortion, 11 weeks, complete complicated by embolism

16. Intrauterine death at 21 weeks gestation, undelivered

17. Normal delivery of single liveborn, 38 weeks; first-degree perineal laceration

18. Inpatient admission: A 33-year-old woman delivered, at 37 weeks, a baby boy weighing 11 lb, 1 oz. Patient had a third degree perineal laceration that was subsequently repaired. The physician indicates that the baby was "large for dates," causing the laceration.

19. Inpatient admission: A grand multipara patient delivers her eighth child at 40 weeks and undergoes a bilateral partial salpingectomy for sterilization. Patient was moderately depressed during her last trimester.

    Discharge diagnoses: Delivery (vaginal) of single liveborn; grand multiparity; depression

20. Inpatient admission: The patient is a 27-year-old female, gravida 2, para 1, admitted at 32 weeks for induced labor due to severe pre-eclampsia and decreased fetal movements. Because of the decreased fetal movements, a cesarean section was performed. She delivered a viable female infant. Postoperatively, the patient was treated with Aldomet and Apresoline for accelerated hypertension.

    Discharge diagnoses: Delivery; severe pre-eclampsia; decreased fetal movements; premature delivery

    Code(s):

Continued

21. Outpatient visit: The patient underwent a cesarean section 10 days prior to this outpatient visit. She presents with an elevated temperature and drainage at the incision site. Hg and Hct are both very low. The physician prescribes iron supplements and antibiotics. A repeat RBC is ordered.

    Impression: Postoperative wound infection

    Code(s):

22. Inpatient admission: The patient was at 31 weeks gestation and was admitted in active labor. Ultrasound revealed that the fetus was in a breech presentation. Although the contractions stopped after three hours, the patient was observed overnight because of her history of being a habitual aborter. Contractions began again on the second day. Because of the obstructed labor, she delivered prematurely a viable infant via cesarean section.

    Discharge diagnoses: Breech delivery; obstructed labor; habitual aborter

    Code(s):

23. Mastitis, four weeks postpartum

24. Supervision of 14-year-old primigravida at 12 weeks gestation

25. Dehiscence of cesarean section wound, five days post-op, seen in physician's office

26. Patient has sprained right ankle; physician states that her pregnancy is not affected by sprain.

27. The 37-year-old elderly primigravida is seen for a regular prenatal visit at 23 weeks gestation.

28. The young patient has pre-existing diabetes mellitus, type 1, seen with ketoacidosis, and arrives at the hospital in a coma. She is at 24 weeks of gestation.

29. The patient is admitted in active labor during week 39 of pregnancy. The patient experienced no complications during her pregnancy. The patient labored for eight hours and delivered a liveborn male over an intact perineum.

30. Premature delivery, 36 weeks, breech presentation obstructing delivery. C-section delivery of a single liveborn female.

31. Encounter at a local family planning clinic for insertion of an intrauterine contraceptive device

32. 29-year-old is admitted for elective sterilization. Patient is experiencing postpartum depression following her last delivery, 12 weeks ago.

33. Intrauterine pregnancy with incompetent cervix, 10 weeks gestation

34. Patient is a 31-year-old woman admitted at 38 weeks for planned C-section. Patient's first delivery was by C-section four years ago. On this admission the patient delivered twin living girls.

35. Intrauterine pregnancy, 20 weeks, dependent on cocaine, seen for prenatal checkup.

36. Delivery of single, stillborn male; patient had severe pre-eclampsia due to pre-existing hypertension. Patient delivered prematurely, at 34 weeks gestation.

37. Twin delivery at 38 weeks with malposition of fetus 1; both liveborn; one placenta and one amniotic sac

38. Outpatient visit: The patient was seen in the prenatal clinic at 30 weeks gestation with pre-existing benign hypertension. The patient reports that she has not felt any fetal movement in several days. The physician could not hear a heartbeat; he performed an ultrasound that revealed a nonviable fetus. Impression: Intrauterine fetal death; hypertension.

39. Outpatient visit: The patient was seen for routine prenatal visit with complaint of hyperemesis. She is a primigravida at 18 weeks gestation and has been unable to eat for several days. Moreover, she has been anemic during the past month. The physician prescribed medication and scheduled a return visit. Impression: Anemia; hyperemesis gravidarum

40. This 25-year-old patient was admitted with difficulty breathing. She has AIDS and is 21 weeks pregnant. Workup reveals *Pneumocystis carinii* pneumonia. What is the correct diagnosis code(s)?

41. The patient, G3P2, was admitted in premature labor at approximately 34 weeks gestation with a history of contractions for the last 24 hours. She was experiencing contractions every five to eight minutes. An ultrasound showed an intrauterine fetal death of triplet 2, but the other two were progressing normally. The contractions stopped for approximately 24 hours, and then started again. It was noted by the physician that the continued contractions were due to fetus 2. The patient was given magnesium sulfate for tocolysis, which was unsuccessful. The patient also developed a fever with an infection of the amniotic sac. The patient continued to be in active labor and due to the infection was allowed to spontaneously deliver the three infants: two liveborn and one fetal death. The patient experienced no postpartum complications. There were multiple amniotic sacs and placentae.

42. Electively induced abortion, complete, complicated by shock, eight weeks gestation

43. Ruptured left tubal pregnancy with hemorrhaging

44. The patient discovered on ultrasound at 11 weeks that the fetus was anencephalic. The mother and father decided to terminate the pregnancy. The patient had an uneventful dilation and curettage.

45. Family planning counseling

46. The new mother develops endometritis one day following a cesarean section delivery (patient is still in the hospital).

Certain Conditions Originating in the Perinatal Period: Congenital Malformations, Deformations, and Chromosomal Abnormalities

OBJECTIVES

After completing this lesson, you should be able to do the following:

- Apply knowledge of current, approved ICD-10-CM coding guidelines to assign and sequence accurate codes for diagnoses related to certain conditions originating in the perinatal period
- Define the perinatal or newborn period
- List Z codes appropriate to use in relation to and conditions in the perinatal period

ICD-10-CM Chapter 16: Certain Conditions Originating in the Perinatal Period (P00–P96)

ICD-10-CM's Chapter 16 includes categories P00–P96 arranged in the following blocks:

P00–P04	Newborn affected by maternal factors and by complications of pregnancy, labor, and delivery
P05–P08	Disorders of newborn related to length of gestation and fetal growth
P09	Abnormal findings on neonatal screening
P10–P15	Birth trauma
P19–P29	Respiratory and cardiovascular disorders specific to the perinatal period
P35–P39	Infections specific to the perinatal period
P50–P61	Hemorrhagic and hematological disorders of newborn

P70–P74	Transitory endocrine and metabolic disorders specific to newborn
P76–P78	Digestive system disorders of newborn
P80–P83	Conditions involving the integument and temperature regulation of newborn
P84	Other problems with newborn
P90–P96	Other disorders originating in the perinatal period

General Coding Guidelines

Codes from this chapter are for use on newborn records only, never on maternal records, and include conditions that have their origin in the fetal or perinatal period (before birth through the first 28 days after birth), even if morbidity occurs later.

Chapter 16 codes may be used throughout the life of the patient if the condition is still present. Codes from this chapter are also applicable only to liveborn infants.

> **EXAMPLE:** A two-month-old seen by a pediatrician is diagnosed with bronchopulmonary dysplasia; the baby was first diagnosed with this condition at age three weeks.
>
> P27.1 Bronchopulmonary dysplasia originating in the perinatal period

> **EXAMPLE:** A 27-year-old woman is diagnosed with vaginal carcinoma due to intrauterine exposure to diethylstilbestrol (DES) taken by her mother during pregnancy.
>
> C52 Malignant neoplasm of the vagina
>
> P04.8 Newborn (suspected to be) affected by other maternal noxious substances

In some instances a newborn has a condition that may be either due to the birth process or community acquired. If the documentation does not indicate which one is appropriate, the default is due to the birth process.

Liveborn Infants According to Place of Birth and Type of Delivery

The birth episode is coded with a code from category Z38, Liveborn infants according to place of birth and type of delivery. ICD-10-CM's Z38 codes specifically identify the number of liveborn infants, where they are born (in hospital, outside hospital), and how they were delivered (vaginally or by cesarean). Other ICD-10-CM codes exist for twin, triplet, quadruplet, quintuplet, and other multiple liveborn infants. For example, the birth record for a single liveborn infant, born in the hospital, and delivered vaginally, is ICD-10-CM code Z38.00. A twin liveborn infant, born in the hospital, and delivered by cesarean, is ICD-10-CM code Z38.31. A code from ICD-10-CM category Z38 is assigned to a newborn once, at the time of birth.

Newborn Affected by Maternal Conditions

Codes P00–P04 are for use when the listed maternal conditions are specified as the cause of confirmed morbidity or potential morbidity, which have their origin in the perinatal period (before birth through the first 28 days after birth). Codes from these categories are also for use for newborns who are suspected of having an abnormal condition resulting from exposure from the mother or the birth process, but without signs or symptoms, and which, after examination and observation, is found not to exist. These codes may be used even if treatment is begun for a suspected condition that is ruled out. Codes from P00–P04 are assigned only when the maternal condition has actually affected the fetus or newborn. The fact that the mother has an associated medical condition or experiences some complication of pregnancy, labor, or delivery does not justify the routine assignment of codes from these categories to the newborn record.

Codes from other chapters may be used along with codes from Chapter 16 if the additional codes from other chapters provide more specific detail.

> **EXAMPLE:** Liveborn infant born (in hospital) with suspected affects from the use of anesthesia during delivery:
>
> Z38.00 Single liveborn, delivered in hospital without mention of cesarean delivery
>
> P04.0 Newborn (suspected) to be affected by maternal anesthesia and analgesia in pregnancy, labor, and delivery
>
> **EXAMPLE:** Delivery of a normal healthy infant (in hospital) to a mother who occasionally uses cocaine:
>
> Z38.00 Single liveborn, delivered in hospital without mention of cesarean delivery

In the first example, the anesthesia use for the delivery was manifested in the infant; therefore, a code from Chapter 16 is assigned. But in the second example, the infant was healthy and normal despite the mother's occasional use of cocaine; therefore, no code is assigned to describe noxious influences of cocaine affecting the fetus (P04.41).

Codes Related to Short Gestation and Low Birth Weight

Codes from category P07, Disorders of newborn related to short gestation and low birth weight, are used for newborns delivered before full term who are defined as either immature or premature.

The definitions used in ICD-10-CM are as follows:

Extremely low birth weight (P07.0-): Newborn birth weight 999 g or less
Other low birth weight newborn (P07.1-): Newborn birth weight 1000–2499 g
Extreme immaturity of newborn (P07.2-): Less than 28 completed weeks (less than 196 completed days) of gestation
Preterm [premature] newborn [other] (P07.3-): 28 completed weeks or more but less than 37 completed weeks (196 completed days but less than 259 completed days) of gestation

Fifth characters indicate specific weights and weeks of gestation. For example, code P07.01 is reported for a newborn of extremely low birth weight of 500 g or less. Code P07.21 is used to report extreme immaturity of a newborn, gestational age of less than 23 completed weeks.

Codes from P07 may be used on subsequent transfers or readmissions; however, the fifth characters for these codes are always based on the original birth weight and not the weight at the subsequent encounter.

Throughout Chapter 16 are notes that help to clarify how codes are to be used. For example, the following note appears under P07: When both birth weight and gestational age of the newborn are available, both should be coded with birth weight sequenced before gestational age.

A code for prematurity should not be assigned unless it is documented. Assignment of codes in categories P05, Disorders of newborn related to slow fetal growth and fetal malnutrition, and P07—Disorders of newborn related to short gestation and low birth weight, not elsewhere classified—should be based on the recorded birth weight and estimated gestational age. Codes from category P05 should not be assigned with codes from category P07.

Codes Related to Long Gestation and High Birth Weight

Category P08 is used to report disorders in the newborn related to long gestation and high birth weight. A note under P08 indicates that when both birth weight and the gestational age of the newborn are available, the birth weight is sequenced first. The following subcategories are included:

- P08.0   Exceptionally large newborn baby (usually implies a birth weight of 4500 g or more)
- P08.1   Other heavy for gestational age newborn (usually implies a birth weight of 4000 to 4499 g)
- P08.2   Late newborn, not heavy for gestational age

These codes are not used for syndrome of infant of diabetic mother or syndrome of infant of mother with gestational diabetes.

Birth Trauma

Codes P10–P15 are used to report birth trauma in newborns. The subcategories in this block include the following:

- P10   Intracranial laceration and hemorrhage due to birth injury
- P11   Other birth injuries to central nervous system
- P12   Birth injury to the scalp
- P13   Birth injury to skeleton
- P14   Birth injury to peripheral nervous system
- P15   Other birth injuries

Fourth characters add more specificity:

- P10.1   Cerebral hemorrhage due to birth injury
- P11.3   Birth injury to facial nerve
- P12.3   Bruising of scalp due to birth injury
- P13.4   Fracture of clavicle due to birth injury
- P14.2   Phrenic nerve paralysis due to birth injury
- P15.5   Birth injury to external genitalia

Respiratory Conditions of Fetus or Newborn

Fetal respiratory conditions are described in the following sections.

Fetal and Newborn Aspiration

Meconium is a newborn's first stool, consisting of a combination of swallowed amniotic fluid and mucus from the baby. The passage of meconium before birth is an indication of fetal distress. It is seen in infants small for gestational age, post dates, or those with cord complications or other factors compromising placental circulation.

Meconium aspiration is defined as the presence of meconium below the vocal cords and occurs in up to 35 percent of the live births with meconium staining. Meconium aspiration syndrome occurs when meconium from amniotic fluid in the upper airway is inhaled in the lungs, which can be fatal. Meconium staining is not meconium aspiration.

Category P24, Neonatal aspiration, describes meconium aspiration and other types of fetal aspiration in the following subcategories or codes:

- P24.0   Meconium aspiration
- P24.1   Neonatal aspiration of (clear) amniotic fluid and mucus
- P24.2   Neonatal aspiration of blood
- P24.3   Neonatal aspiration of milk and regurgitated food
- P24.8   Other neonatal aspiration
- P24.9   Neonatal aspiration, unspecified

The fifth characters in the above codes identify the presence or absence of respiratory symptoms. Code P24.01 is also used for the term *massive meconium aspiration*, even though it is somewhat different from meconium aspiration.

Meconium ileus and meconium plug syndrome are reported with code P76.0, Meconium plug syndrome. The exception to this is when meconium plug syndrome is associated with cystic fibrosis, in which case code E84.11 is assigned.

Fetal Respiratory Distress and Asphyxia

Fetal distress usually refers to metabolic abnormalities, such as hypoxia and acidosis, which may lead to failure of vital organs and ultimately to permanent injury or death. Code P19 is used to describe metabolic acidemia in a newborn with fourth characters, which indicate when the acidemia occurred. For example, P19.1 is used to report metabolic acidemia in a newborn first noted during labor.

Other Respiratory Conditions

Category P28 describes several respiratory conditions originating in the perinatal period. Some examples include the following:

- P28.0   Primary atelectasis of newborn
- P28.2   Cyanotic attacks of newborn
- P28.3   Primary sleep apnea of newborn
- P28.5   Respiratory failure of newborn

Bacterial Sepsis of Newborn

If a newborn is documented as having sepsis without documentation of congenital or community acquired, the default is congenital, and a code from category P36 should be assigned. If the P36 code includes the causal organism, an additional code from category B95—*Streptococcus*, *Staphylococcus*, and *Enterococcus* as the cause of diseases classified elsewhere—or B96, Other bacterial agents as the cause of diseases classified elsewhere, should not be assigned. If the P36 code does not include the causal organism, assign an additional code from category B96. If applicable, use additional codes to identify severe sepsis (R65.2-) and any associated acute organ dysfunction.

Hemolytic Disease of the Newborn

Category P55 is used to describe hemolytic disease in newborns due to either Rh isoimmunization or ABO isoimmunization. Code P55.9 is used to describe other hemolytic disease of newborns. The coding of this condition is based on physician documentation after routine cord blood testing.

Apparent Life-Threatening Event

Code R68.13, Apparent life-threatening event in infant, is assigned to a documented life-threatening event. This was previously referred to as near miss sudden infant death syndrome.

Necrotizing Enterocolitis

Necrotizing enterocolitis is a condition that is seen primarily in premature infants. Portions of the intestines undergo necrosis or death of the tissue. It is a major cause of illness and death in these premature infants. Symptoms include feeding intolerance, abdominal distension, and bloody stools. The condition usually progresses to intestinal peritonitis, perforation, and general hypotension.

Code P77 is used to describe the three stages of necrotizing enterocolitis. Stage one (P77.1) describes necrotizing enterocolitis without pneumatosis or perforation. Stage two (P77.2) describes necrotizing enterocolitis with pneumatosis but without perforation. Stage three describes necrotizing enterocolitis with pneumatosis and perforation.

Observation and Evaluation of Newborns and Infants

A code from categories P00–P04 is assigned when a healthy newborn or infant is evaluated for a suspected condition, without signs or symptoms, that is found not to be present when the study is completed. When assigned on the same admission as the birth of the newborn, a code from P00–P04 is assigned as an additional code. It may be assigned as the principal diagnosis for a later encounter or readmission after the birth of the infant. It is used only for the first 28 days of life.

Stillbirth

Code P95, Stillbirth, is only for use in institutions that maintain separate records for stillbirths. No other code should be used with P95. Code P95 is not to be used on the mother's record.

Z Codes Used for Infants and Newborns

Subcategory code Z00.1 is used to report encounters for newborn health examinations. These codes are used for children under 29 days. Fifth characters differentiate between health examination for newborns under 8 days (Z00.110) and health examination for newborn 8 to 28 days (Z00.111). Code Z00.121 is used for encounters for routine child health exams (children over 28 days) with abnormal findings. Code Z00.129 is used for encounters for routine child health exams without abnormal findings.

Code Z23 is used when a child presents for immunizations. A code from subcategory Z00.1—Encounter for newborn, infant, and child health examinations—is assigned for well-baby checks of infants and children when there is no problem identified. The codes are based on the age of the patient; that is, under 8 days, 8 to 28 days, and over 28 days.

ICD-10-CM Chapter 17: Congenital Malformations, Deformations, and Chromosomal Abnormalities

The newborn period begins at birth and lasts through the 28th day following birth. All clinically significant conditions noted on routine newborn examination should be coded. A condition is significant when it requires any of the following:

- Clinical evaluation
- Therapeutic treatment
- Diagnostic procedures
- Extended length of hospital stay
- Increased nursing care or monitoring
- Implications for the future healthcare needs of the child

The preceding guidelines are identical to the general coding guidelines for selection of other diagnoses, with the exception of the final item regarding implications for future healthcare needs. Only the physician can determine whether a condition is clinically significant. Pediatricians or neonatologists generally treat newborns and infants.

Chapter 17 of ICD-10-CM includes categories Q00–Q99 arranged in the following blocks:

- Q00–Q07   Congenital malformations of the nervous system
- Q10–Q18   Congenital malformations of eye, ear, face, and neck
- Q20–Q28   Congenital malformations of the circulatory system
- Q30–Q34   Congenital malformations of the respiratory system
- Q35–Q37   Cleft lip and cleft palate
- Q38–Q45   Other congenital malformations of the digestive system
- Q50–Q56   Congenital malformations of genital organs
- Q60–Q64   Congenital malformations of the urinary system
- Q65–Q79   Congenital malformations and deformations of the musculoskeletal system
- Q80–Q89   Other congenital malformations
- Q90–Q99   Chromosomal abnormalities, not elsewhere classified

Coding Guidelines and Instructional Notes

Codes from Chapter 17 may be used throughout the life of the patient, as long as the condition is present; the condition is not only coded at birth or when it is first diagnosed. If a congenital malformation or deformity has been corrected, a personal history code should be used to identify the history of the malformation or deformity.

Conditions included in Chapter 17 are organized by body system—for example, Q20–Q28, Congenital malformations of the circulatory system, and Q65–Q79, Congenital malformations and deformations of the musculoskeletal system—and include laterality for limbs and bones.

These codes are assigned when a malformation or deformation or chromosomal abnormality is documented, and the code may be the principal or first listed diagnosis on a record or a secondary diagnosis.

When no unique code is available, assign additional code(s) for any manifestations that may be present. When the code assignment specifically identifies the malformation, deformation, or chromosomal abnormality, manifestations that are an inherent component of the anomaly should not be coded separately. Additional codes should be assigned for manifestations that are not an inherent component.

For the birth admission, the appropriate code from category Z38, Liveborn infants, according to place of birth and type of delivery, should be sequenced as the principal diagnosis, followed by any congenital anomaly codes, Q00–Q89.

If a congenital anomaly is noted during the hospital admission when the infant is born, the code describing the anomaly is assigned as an additional diagnosis. The principal diagnosis is a code from the category Z38, Liveborn infants according to type of birth.

> **EXAMPLE:** Liveborn male infant born in the hospital with Tetralogy of Fallot:
>
> Z38.00 Single liveborn, delivered in hospital without mention of cesarean delivery
>
> Q21.3 Tetralogy of Fallot

However, if the infant was transferred on the day of birth to another hospital for care of the congenital anomaly, the principal diagnosis at the second hospital would be the congenital anomaly.

> **EXAMPLE:** Liveborn male infant transferred for care of thoracic spina bifida with hydrocephalus:
>
> Q05.1 Spina bifida of dorsal [thoracic] region with hydrocephalus

The following subsections describe several common congenital anomalies.

Spina Bifida

Spina bifida is a defective closure of the vertebral column. It ranges in severity from the occult type, revealing few signs, to a completely open spine (rachischisis). In spina bifida cystica, the protruding sac contains meninges (meningocele), the spinal cord (myelocele), or both (myelomeningocele). Commonly seen in the lumbar, low thoracic, or sacral region, spina bifida extends for three to six vertebral segments. When the spinal cord or lumbosacral nerve roots are involved in the spina bifida, as is usually the case, varying degrees of paralysis occur below the involved level. The result may be orthopedic conditions, such as clubfoot or dislocated hip. The paralysis usually affects the sphincters of the bladder and rectum. Hydrocephalus, an excessive accumulation of cerebrospinal fluid within the ventricles, is associated with at least 80 percent of the lumbosacral type.

Code Q05 is used to report spina bifida, with fourth characters describing the portion of the spine affected. These codes also differentiate between spina bifida with and without hydrocephalus. The coder is instructed to use an additional code for any associated paraplegia.

Cardiac Conditions

Congenital heart defects can be divided into two types: cyanotic and acyanotic. Acyanotic defects continue to eject oxygenated blood from the heart. The following conditions are classified as acyanotic:

- Aortic stenosis (AS)
- Atrial septal defect (ASD)
- Coarctation of the aorta
- Endocardial cushion defect

- Patent ductus arteriosus (PDA)
- Pulmonary stenosis (PS)
- Ventricular septal defect (VSD)

Cyanotic heart defects allow right-to-left shunting of unoxygenated blood that mixes with oxygenated blood, resulting in arterial blood oxygen desaturation. The following defects are considered cyanotic:

- Hypoplastic left ventricle syndrome
- Hypoplastic right ventricle syndrome
- Persistent truncus arteriosus (PTA)
- Pulmonary atresia
- Tetralogy of Fallot (TOF)
- Total anomalous pulmonary venous return (TAPVR)
- Complete transposition of great vessels (TGV)
- Tricuspid atresia

Two of the most common congenital cardiac defects are ventricular septal defect and patent ductus arteriosus. Ventricular septal defect, the more common of the two, is an abnormal communication or opening in the ventricular septum that allows the blood to shunt from the left ventricle to the right ventricle. The defect may be small or large and can occur in several locations in the heart, most commonly in the area of the membranous septum. Although some of the smaller asymptomatic defects close spontaneously in some people by the age of seven or eight years, others will require corrective surgery. In repair, a prosthetic material of Dacron or Teflon is used to patch the defect. ICD-10-CM classifies septal defects to code Q21.

In patent ductus arteriosus, the fetal blood vessel that connects the aorta and the pulmonary artery, the ductus arteriosus, allows blood to bypass nonfunctioning fetal lungs. Within the first 72 hours of life, the ductus arteriosus begins to constrict, and within 12 weeks, it completely closes. In some patients, especially premature infants with respiratory distress syndrome, the ductus arteriosus does not close. When the ductus arteriosus remains open, heart failure and pulmonary congestion result. When surgical repair is required, ligation of the ductus arteriosus is performed. ICD-10-CM assigns code Q25.0 for patent ductus arteriosus.

Cleft Lip and Cleft Palate

Cleft lip, cleft palate, and combinations of the two are the most common congenital anomalies of the head and neck. A cleft is characterized by a fissure or elongated opening of a specified site, usually forming during the embryonic stage. Cleft lips and palates are classified as partial or complete and can occur either bilaterally or unilaterally. The most common clefts are left unilateral complete clefts of the primary and secondary palate, and partial midline clefts of the secondary palate involving the soft palate and part of the hard palate. The incisive foramen serves as the dividing point between the primary and secondary palates.

In ICD-10-CM, cleft palate and cleft lip are classified to categories Q35–Q37. Subcategory codes under code Q35 identify which part of the palate is involved; for example, Q35.1, Cleft hard palate; Q35.3, Cleft soft palate; and Q35.7, Cleft uvula.

Fourth characters under code Q36, Cleft lip, identify whether the condition is bilateral (Q36.0), median (Q36.1), or unilateral (Q36.9).

Subcategory Q37 is used to report the condition of cleft palate with cleft lip, with the fourth characters differentiating among the various types.

Pyloric Stenosis

Pyloric stenosis results from hypertrophy of the circular and longitudinal muscularis of the pylorus and distal antrum of the stomach. In this case, the infant typically feeds well until about two weeks after birth, at which time regurgitation of food occasionally occurs. Several days later, projectile vomiting begins. Dehydration due to the vomiting is common. Surgery is the preferred treatment. Fredet-Ramstedt pyloromyotomy is performed after the dehydration has been managed. Congenital or infantile pyloric stenosis is assigned code Q40.0.

Uterine Anomalies

The development of the female reproductive tract is a complex process that involves a highly orchestrated series of events including cellular, differentiation, migration, fusion, and canalization. Failure of any part of the process results in congenital anomalies. The American Society of Reproductive Medicine has identified several types of uterine, cervical, and vaginal anomalies, many of which are classified to category Q51:

- Q51.0   Agenesis and aplasia of uterus
- Q51.1   Doubling of uterus with doubling of cervix and vagina
- Q51.2   Other doubling of uterus
- Q51.3   Bicornate uterus
- Q51.4   Unicornate uterus
- Q51.5   Agenesis and aplasia of cervix
- Q51.6   Embryonic cyst of cervix
- Q51.7   Congenital fistulae between uterus and digestive and urinary tracts
- Q51.8   Other congenital malformations of uterus and cervix

Other Malformations of Genital Organs

Congenital malformations of genital organs of infant males are classified to categories Q53 through Q55. Conditions classified to these categories include undescended and ectopic testis, hypospadias, and other abnormalities of the scrotum and penis. Examples of codes include the following:

- Q53.01   Ectopic testis, unilateral
- Q53.02   Ectopic testis, bilateral
- Q53.11   Abdominal testis, unilateral
- Q54.0   Hypospadias, balanic
- Q54.1   Hypospadias, penile
- Q55.21   Polyorchism
- Q55.3   Atresia of vas deferens
- Q55.5   Congenital absence and aplasia of penis
- Q55.64   Hidden penis

ICD-10-CM also provides code Q56, Indeterminate sex and pseudohermaphroditism, which distinguishes between male and female pseudohermaphroditism.

Polycystic Kidney Disease

Polycystic kidney disease is an inherited disorder characterized by multiple, bilateral, grapelike clusters of fluid-filled cysts that grossly enlarge the kidneys, compressing and eventually replacing functioning renal tissue. The infantile form of this condition reveals an infant with pronounced epicanthal folds, a pointed nose, a small chin, and floppy, low-set ears. Signs of respiratory distress and congestive heart failure also may be present. This condition eventually deteriorates into uremia and renal failure. ICD-10-CM classifies polycystic kidney, infantile type, to Q61.1 and polycystic kidney, adult type, to Q61.2.

When there is no further specification as to the type of polycystic kidney disease, code Q61.3 should be assigned.

Chapter 17: ICD-10-CM Exercises

Review the following statements and cases and assign the appropriate codes:

1. Single liveborn male (born in the hospital via cesarean delivery) with congenital diaphragmatic hernia

2. Single liveborn male (normal delivery), with polydactyly of fingers

3. Physician's office visit: unilateral cleft lip and hard palate

4. Physician's office visit: congenital talipes equinovalgus; Down syndrome

5. Twin male (male liveborn) born in hospital via cesarean section; bilateral cryptorchism

6. Physician's office visit: hypoglycemia in infant born of diabetic mother

7. Physician's office visit: patent ductus arteriosus

8. Single liveborn (born in hospital via vaginal delivery); erythroblastosis fetalis due to ABO incompatibility

9. Single liveborn male (born in hospital via vaginal delivery); premature at 29 weeks (1300 g); hyaline membrane disease

10. Single liveborn male (born in hospital via vaginal delivery); necrotizing enterocolitis, stage 1, discovered in a newborn at birth

11. Single liveborn (female) born on the way to the hospital but admitted directly to the newborn nursery

12. Two-year-old diagnosed with fragile X syndrome

Continued

13. Term birth, single female, with partial facial paralysis, vaginal delivery

14. Physician's office visit: The patient is a three-month-old girl who was seen for an evaluation of a right clubfoot. She is currently asymptomatic but tests positive for HIV.

    Impression: Talipes equinovarus; positive for HIV
    Code(s):

15. Inpatient admission: The baby girl was born prematurely by cesarean section at 31 weeks and 1900 g. She was found to have a coarctation of aorta. Prior to corrective surgery, the infant developed respiratory distress and was subsequently intubated. Her condition improved, and she was discharged on the sixth hospital day after delivery.

    Discharge diagnoses: Prematurity; coarctation of aorta; respiratory distress
    Code(s):

16. Inpatient admission: The six-week-old infant was admitted to the emergency department with a 48-hour history of upper respiratory infection. The baby had been crying for several hours. Examination revealed acute suppurative otitis media and upper respiratory infection. The baby had been seeing the pediatrician weekly for failure to thrive. The baby was started on antibiotics and admitted.

    Discharge diagnoses: Bilateral acute suppurative otitis media; upper respiratory infection; failure to thrive
    Code(s):

17. Inpatient admission: The infant patient was born in the hospital to a 23-year-old primigravida. When induction of labor failed, the baby was delivered by cesarean section. The mother was a known chronic alcoholic; therefore, the newborn was placed in the neonatal intensive care unit for observation for possible alcohol-related problems. The baby appeared to be fine.

    Discharge diagnosis: Single newborn
    Code(s):

18. Cephalhematoma due to birth injury one week ago; physician continues to monitor baby in case further treatment is needed.

19. Full-term newborn was delivered four days ago and discharged home. The infant was readmitted to the hospital and diagnosed with hyperbilirubinemia. Phototherapy was initiated, and the baby will continue to have phototherapy provided at home after discharge.

20. Full-term female infant was born in this hospital by vaginal delivery. Her mother has been an alcoholic for many years and would not stop drinking during her pregnancy. The baby was born with fetal alcohol syndrome and was placed in the NICU.

21. Premature baby born in the hospital by cesarean section to a mother dependent on cocaine. The newborn did not show signs of withdrawal. Birth weight of 1247 g; 31 completed weeks of gestation. Dehydration was also diagnosed and treated.

22. Stage 3 necrotizing enterocolitis in newborn; baby was transferred from a local acute care hospital.

23. Mother was concerned about urinary output and brought the baby in for an examination. Abdominal ultrasound in physician's office indicates that the three-month-old has an accessory kidney.

24. Newborn is diagnosed with ventricular septal defect, pulmonary stenosis, dextroposition of aorta, and hypertrophy of right ventricle. The physician documents as final diagnosis Tetralogy of Fallot.

25. Atresia of esophagus with tracheoesophageal fistula

26. Newborn born in the community hospital transferred to a specialty hospital for treatment for hypoplastic left heart syndrome. Code for the specialty hospital.

27. A 25-year-old male was admitted for a heart valve replacement for aortic insufficiency. The patient's condition was secondary to his Marfan syndrome.

28. Congenital bilateral hip dislocation

29. A 43-year-old woman is admitted for treatment of vaginal carcinoma. Her physician documents DES use by the patient's mother during pregnancy.

30. Meconium aspiration syndrome in newborn male with nuchal cord compression, born by vaginal delivery

31. Transferred from hospital A to hospital B with spina bifida involving the dorsal region with hydrocephalus; code for hospital B.

32. Newborn (born in hospital) via normal spontaneous vaginal delivery with respiratory failure

33. Routine well baby visit for six-week-old baby girl

34. Physician's office visit for one-year-old infant with childhood polycystic disease

35. The patient is the oldest of triplets delivered at 34 weeks' gestation. The baby was 2200 g and generally in good health. He was on supplemental oxygen for one day (as were his siblings) for transient tachypnea. The newborn received the oxygen by CPAP and did well. By the second day, the baby was weaned from the supplemental oxygen and was breathing completely on his own.

Symptoms, Signs, and Abnormal Clinical and Laboratory Findings

OBJECTIVES

After completing this lesson, you should be able to do the following:

- Apply knowledge of current ICD-10-CM coding guidelines to assign and sequence accurate codes for diagnoses related to signs, symptoms, and ill-defined conditions
- Differentiate between a sign and a symptom
- Identify conditions that are integral to a disease process and those that are not
- Recognize the most common signs and symptoms

ICD-10-CM

Chapter 18 of the ICD-10-CM code book, Symptoms, signs and abnormal clinical and laboratory findings, is divided into the following sections. The codes in these sections, like all ICD-10-CM codes, may be used by physicians of any medical specialty or by general practitioners.

The following blocks represent the ICD-10-CM codes for Chapter 18, symptoms, signs and abnormal clinical and laboratory findings, not elsewhere classified (R00–R99):

R00–R09	Symptoms and signs involving the circulatory and respiratory systems
R10–R19	Symptoms and signs involving the digestive system and abdomen
R20–R23	Symptoms and signs involving the skin and subcutaneous tissue
R25–R29	Symptoms and signs involving the nervous and musculoskeletal systems
R30–R39	Symptoms and signs involving the genitourinary system
R40–R46	Symptoms and signs involving cognition, perception, emotional state and behavior
R47–R49	Symptoms and signs involving speech and voice
R50–R69	General symptoms and signs
R70–R79	Abnormal findings on examination of blood, without diagnosis
R80–R82	Abnormal findings on examination of urine, without diagnosis
R83–R89	Abnormal findings on examination of other body fluids, substances and tissues, without diagnosis

R90–R94   Abnormal findings on diagnostic imaging and in function studies, without diagnosis

R97   Abnormal tumor markers

R99   Ill-defined and unknown cause of mortality

A sign is objective evidence of a disease observed by a physician. A symptom is any subjective evidence of disease reported by the patient to the physician. It should be noted that the symptoms associated with a given organ system are classified to that particular chapter in the code book. Signs and symptoms that can apply to more than one disease or system, or those of undetermined etiology can be found In Chapter 18.

Symptoms and Signs

Categories R00–R69 include a variety of symptoms, many of which are appropriately reported as additional diagnoses. The signs and symptoms described in these categories are used when the following occur:

- Cases exist for which no more specific diagnosis can be made, even after all the facts bearing on the cases have been investigated.

- Signs or symptoms existing at the time of the initial encounter prove to be transient, and their causes cannot be determined.

- Provisional diagnoses remain for a patient who fails to return for further investigation or care.

- Cases are referred elsewhere for investigation or treatment, before the diagnosis is made.

- A more precise diagnosis is unavailable for any other reason.

- Certain symptoms represent important problems in medical care, and it might be desirable to classify them in addition to a known cause.

- A symptom that was treated in an outpatient setting did not have the workup necessary to determine a definitive diagnosis.

- A residual sequelae is the actual reason for admission, and the Alphabetic Index. Directs the coder to the appropriate code.

Symptoms and signs are used frequently to describe reasons for service in outpatient settings. Outpatient visits do not always allow for the type of study that is needed to determine a diagnosis. Often the purpose of the outpatient visit is to relieve the symptom rather than to determine or treat the underlying condition. Coders must code the outpatient's condition to the highest level of certainty. The highest level of certainty is often an abnormal sign or symptom code that is assigned as the reason for the outpatient visit.

Although symptom codes are usually not designated as a principal diagnosis when a specific condition has already been identified, a symptom can be the principal diagnosis when the patient encounter is for treating the symptom, and no further treatment or evaluation takes place.

Nonspecific Abnormal Findings on Laboratory, X-ray, Pathologic, and Other Diagnostic Tests

Categories R70–R94 include codes for nonspecific abnormal findings on laboratory, x-ray, pathologic, and other diagnostic tests. In the outpatient setting, these codes may provide further explanation of the service provided, such as an elevated blood pressure reading (R03.0) that requires further monitoring and workup.

The following guidelines apply when nonspecific abnormal findings in the inpatient setting are coded:

- Abnormal findings from laboratory, x-ray, pathologic, and other diagnostic results are not coded and reported, unless the physician indicates their clinical significance. When the findings are outside the normal range, and the physician has ordered other tests to evaluate the condition or has prescribed treatment, it is appropriate to ask the physician whether the diagnosis code(s) for the abnormal findings should be added.

- Notes in the section on abnormal clinical and laboratory findings direct coders to search elsewhere in the ICD-10-CM code book when documentation in the health record states the presence of a specific condition. Codes for these specific conditions are located in the Alphabetic Index under Findings, abnormal, without diagnosis.

Often abnormal findings are the reason for additional testing to be performed on patients in the outpatient setting. For example, elevated levels of prostate specific antigen (PSA), R97.2, may be a reason for continued testing or monitoring of a patient. The code does not provide a specific diagnosis but instead indicates an abnormal finding for a specific organ. Abnormal findings that are documented in the record may or may not be appropriate to code. When the coder notes an abnormal laboratory finding that appears to have triggered additional testing or therapy, the physician should be asked whether the abnormal finding is a clinically significant condition.

The radiologist's findings can be used to identify the specific site of a fracture when the physician's diagnosis statement is nonspecific. For example, the attending physician writes "Fracture, left tibia." However, the radiologist describes the injury as a fracture of the shaft of the tibia. The coder may code "fracture, tibia, shaft," based on the specific findings by the radiologist.

The radiologist's findings also may be used to clarify an outpatient's diagnosis or reason for services. For example, a patient comes to the hospital for an outpatient x-ray. The physician's order for the x-ray is "possible kidney stones." The radiologist's statement on the radiology report is "bilateral nephrolithiasis." Because the radiologist is a physician, it is appropriate to code calculus of the kidney as the patient's diagnosis.

Ill-Defined and Unknown Causes of Mortality

Category R99, Ill-defined and unknown causes of mortality, includes conditions for which further specification is not provided in the health record or for which the underlying cause is unknown.

Common Signs and Symptoms

As previously discussed, when symptoms are routinely associated with a particular condition, only that condition is reported. However, when the symptom is not routinely associated with a specific condition, two separate codes may be assigned.

Some of the most common signs and symptoms are listed here:

Syncope (R55): Syncope is a fainting spell that usually follows a feeling of lightheadedness and may be prevented either by lying down or by sitting with the head between the knees. It may be caused by many different factors, including emotional stress, pooling of blood in the legs, heavy sweating, or a sudden change in room temperature or body position. Code R55 may be assigned when the diagnostic statement indicates blackout, fainting, or vasovagal attack.

Convulsions (R56): Convulsions are characterized by a sudden, violent, and uncontrollable contraction of a group of muscles. Convulsions and seizures designated as febrile, not otherwise specified, are assigned code R56.0-; complex febrile convulsions are reported with R56.01; posttraumatic are identified with code R56.1; and all other unspecific seizures or convulsions are assigned code R56.9.

Dizziness and giddiness (R42): This condition is a feeling of faintness or an inability to keep normal balance in a standing or a seated position. It sometimes is linked to mental confusion, nausea, and weakness. Code R42 also may be assigned when the diagnostic statement indicates lightheadedness, vertigo, or giddiness.

Early satiety (R68.81): Early satiety is common in many conditions, such as hormone problems or a brain tumor. It is not the same as anorexia. Early satiety occurs in persons who have hunger and are eating but feel full.

Facial weakness (R29.810): This code is used when facial weakness is not a sequelae of a cerebrovascular accident.

Disturbance of skin sensation (R20.-): This condition describes the loss of skin sensation, often associated with tingling. It is assigned when the documentation states anesthesia of the skin, burning or prickling sensation of the skin, hyperesthesia or hypoesthesia of the skin, numbness, paresthesia, or tingling of the skin.

Abnormal weight loss or underweight (R63.4 and R63.6): A relatively recent weight loss is reported with code R63.4, whereas the condition of weighing less than a person's standard weight for height is reported with code R63.6. The coder is instructed to also identify the body mass index (Z68.-) if it is known.

Lack of expected normal physiological development in childhood (R62.50): Fifth character codes in this subcategory describe three distinctive conditions relating to developmental problems. Failure to thrive, R62.51, is a condition where infants or children lose weight or fail to gain weight in accordance with standardized growth charts. Short stature, R62.52, is a diagnosis for a slower than normal rate of maturation. Code R62.50 simply refers to an unspecified lack of expected normal physiological development.

Epistaxis (R04.0): Epistaxis is a nosebleed caused by irritation of the soft inner lining of the nose, violent sneezing, or fragile arteries in the nose. Additionally, it may be caused by long-term infection, injury, high blood pressure, leukemia, or lack of vitamin K. Epistaxis may result from tiny blood vessels breaking in the wall between the nostrils (nasal septum). It often occurs in children. In adults, it is more common among men than women and may be severe in elderly persons. Epistaxis may cause respiratory distress, dizziness, and nausea, and blood loss may lead to fainting.

Palpitations (R00.2): Palpitations are characterized by a pounding or racing of the heart and are linked to normal emotional responses or with some heart disorders. Some people may complain of a pounding heart and show no sign of heart disease. Others, who have serious heart disorders, may not detect palpitations. When the palpitations occur as a result of an established condition, such as atrial fibrillation, the palpitation code is not reported.

Enlargement of lymph nodes (R59.5): Enlargement of lymph nodes also is referred to as lymphadenopathy or swollen glands. Code R59.5 is reported when a definitive diagnosis has not been established.

Hyperventilation (R06.4): Hyperventilation is characterized by a breathing rate that is greater than that necessary for the exchange of oxygen and carbon dioxide. Its causes include asthma or early emphysema; increased metabolism because of exercise, fever, hyperthyroidism, or infections; damage to the central nervous system, as in cerebral thrombosis; encephalitis, head injuries, or meningitis; certain hormones and drugs; difficulties with mechanical respirators; and mental factors such as anxiety and pain.

Nausea with vomiting (R11.2): This category refers to a common stomach upset. However, when the condition is documented as vomiting of blood (hematemesis), code K92.0 should be assigned.

Heartburn (R12): Heartburn is a painful, burning sensation in the throat (esophagus) just below the breastbone. Typically, heartburn is caused by stomach contents flowing back into the esophagus, but it also may be caused by too much acid in the stomach or by a peptic ulcer.

Dysphagia (R13.10): Dysphagia is difficulty in swallowing, commonly linked to blockage or motor disorders of the esophagus. Patients with blockages such as esophageal tumors or lower esophageal rings are unable to swallow solids but can tolerate liquids.

Diarrhea (R19.7): Usually, diarrhea is a symptom of some other disorder or of a more severe disease, in which case it should not be coded separately. It may be accompanied by vomiting and various other symptoms that should be coded when present.

Retention of urine (R33.9): This is the abnormal accumulation of urine in the bladder due to the inability to urinate.

Incontinence of urine (R32): This is the inability to completely control urination with involuntary passage of urine.

Abdominal pain, unspecified (R10.9): This is abdominal pain unspecified as to cause and site of pain.

Outpatient Coding Guidelines

Many outpatient visits are coded with ICD-10-CM codes for signs and symptoms when a definitive diagnosis has not been established. Coders of outpatient visits must follow Section IV: Diagnostic coding and reporting guidelines for outpatient services, within the ICD-10-CM Official Guidelines for Coding and Reporting.

Signs, symptoms, abnormal test results, or other reasons for the outpatient visit are used when a physician qualifies a diagnostic statement using terms indicating uncertainty such as, possible, probable, suspected, questionable, rule out, working diagnosis. The condition qualified in that statement should not be coded as if it existed. Rather, the condition should be coded to the highest degree of certainty, such as the signs or symptoms the patient exhibits. For example, the physician writes the diagnosis for an outpatient as "rule out pneumonia" and describes the patient as having fever, cough, and malaise. Pneumonia is not coded for this patient. Instead, the symptoms of fever, cough, and malaise are coded, as this is what is known as certain to be occurring in the patient. Pneumonia has not been confirmed.

These guidelines differ from acute care, short-term, long-term, and psychiatric hospital inpatient rules, where a qualified condition is coded as if it exists, because the evaluation and management of the suspected condition in these settings is often equal to the treatment of the same condition that has been confirmed.

The term *ruled out* designates that the condition stated to be ruled out does not exist. This condition, therefore, cannot be coded, and the preceding signs, symptoms, or abnormal test results are coded instead.

Glasgow Coma Scale

Something new for ICD-10-CM is the incorporation of the Glasgow coma scale (codes R40.211–R40.236). The Glasgow coma scale is for use with codes for traumatic brain injury or sequelae of cerebrovascular disease codes. Although these codes may be used in any setting, they are primarily used by trauma registries and for research. The Glasgow coma scale codes are to be sequenced after the diagnosis code(s). These codes (R40.21, eyes open; R40.22, best verbal response; and R40.23, best motor response) are all needed to complete the scale. The various seventh characters indicate when the scale was recorded, and the character should match for all three codes. The seventh characters areas follows:

0—unspecified time
1—in the field [EMT or ambulance]
2—at arrival to emergency department
3—at hospital admission
4—24 hours or more after hospital admission

Code R40.24, Glasgow coma scale, total score, is also a part of the Glasgow coma scale and it is used when only a total score is documented instead of all the levels being listed out separately. At a minimum, report the initial score documented on presentation at the facility.

Chapter 18: ICD-10-CM Exercises

Review the following statements and cases and assign the appropriate codes:

1. Right lower quadrant abdominal pain

2. Abnormal mammogram

3. Ten-month-old infant with excessive crying, fever, and runny nose; final diagnoses: acute rhinitis and acute left otitis media

4. Abnormal glandular Pap smear of the cervix

5. Shortness of breath, cause undetermined

6. Shock

7. Pneumonia with cough

8. Office visit: rule out diabetes; patient complains of polydipsia and polyuria for four weeks prior to visit.

9. Stress urinary incontinence in male patient

10. Seizures; epilepsy, ruled out

11. Abdominal mass with jaundice

12. Abnormal glucose tolerance test

13. Elevated PSA

14. Failure to thrive in two-year-old child

15. A male patient was admitted to the hospital because of severe anterior mid-sternal chest pain also involving both arms. Several cardiac procedures were performed (heart catheterization, arteriography, and angiography), but they revealed no coronary artery disease. The patient's pain improved, and he was discharged in no apparent distress.

    Discharge diagnosis: Chest pain with no coronary artery disease

    Code(s):

16. A 43-year-old female patient was seen in the emergency department with generalized abdominal pain that was moderate to severe in intensity. Blood work showed an elevated white blood count. The diagnosis at the time the patient was seen was thought to be possible acute cholecystitis. Several tests were run (intravenous pyelogram, cholecystogram, and gallbladder ultrasound), all of which came back within normal limits. Within a couple of days, the patient became pain free, her white count returned to normal, and she asked to leave the hospital, because she was feeling better.

    Discharge diagnoses: Abdominal pain; leukocytosis

    Code(s):

17. Chronic fatigue syndrome

18. Concentration deficit

19. Non-visualization of gallbladder on x-ray examination; the x-ray exam is not coded.

20. Respiratory arrest of unknown origin

21. Acute idiopathic pulmonary hemorrhage diagnosed in a two-month old baby

22. Abnormality of gait

23. Outpatient encounter to change a patient's surgical dressing

24. Right upper quadrant rebound abdominal tenderness

25. An ENT physician sees a male patient in the office because of a bad nosebleed. Upon questioning the patient, the physician discovered that he was prone to nosebleeds, but this one was particularly bad. The physician packed the nose and diagnosed recurrent epistaxis. What diagnosis would be coded?

26. Sinoatrial bradycardia

27. Patient is experiencing extreme fatigue following her chemotherapy treatment three days ago. She states that "she is so tired she can hardly get out of bed." She had right breast carcinoma previously excised. How would this be coded?

28. Sudden infant death syndrome (SIDS)

Injury, Poisonings, and Adverse Effects

ICD-10-CM

Chapter 19 of the ICD-10-CM code book covers a wide variety of injuries and includes subsections on poisonings, adverse effects of drugs, and complications of surgical and medical care. Physicians of many specialties use codes from this chapter. Certainly, emergency department physicians and orthopedists use many of the fracture and other injury codes, but general practitioners and internists also use many of the codes from the adverse effects and poisoning sections. In addition, physicians of many specialties, including dermatologists, general practitioners, and internists, may treat patients with burns.

Codes in ICD-10-CM are arranged by body part. The blocks relating to injuries include the following:

S00–S09	Injuries to the head
S10–S19	Injuries to the neck
S20–S29	Injuries to the thorax
S30–S39	Injuries to the abdomen, lower back, lumbar spine, pelvis and external genitals
S40–S49	Injuries to the shoulder and upper arm
S50–S59	Injuries to the elbow and forearm
S60–S69	Injuries to the wrist, hand and fingers
S70–S79	Injuries to the hip and thigh
S80–S89	Injuries to the knee and lower leg
S90–S99	Injuries to the ankle and foot
T07	Injuries involving multiple body regions
T14	Injury of unspecified body region
T15–T19	Effects of foreign body entering through natural orifice
T20–T32	Burns and corrosions
T33–T34	Frostbite
T36–T50	Poisoning by, adverse effect of and underdosing of drugs, medicaments and biological substances
T51–T65	Toxic effects of substances chiefly nonmedicinal as to source
T66–T78	Other and unspecified effects of external causes
T79	Certain early complications of trauma
T80–T88	Complications of surgical and medical care, not elsewhere classified

Within each block the injuries are arranged in the following order:

- Superficial injury
- Open wound
- Fracture
- Dislocation and sprain
- Injury of nerves
- Injury of blood vessels
- Injury of muscle and tendon
- Crushing injury
- Traumatic amputation
- Other and unspecified injuries

The terms *displaced* and *nondisplaced* are new in ICD-10-CM as is the term *corrosion*. Corrosions are burns that are due to chemicals versus those due to a heat source, electricity, or radiation. Finally, the concept of underdosing is introduced in ICD-10-CM. These will be discussed later in the chapter.

Injuries

Injuries are traumatic in nature and result in damage to body parts, which may result in tissue death. Various external causes such as a blow, a fall, a gun, a knife, industrial equipment, or a household item may be responsible for an injury. Moreover, traumatic injuries may predispose a person to a nontraumatic disease. For example, bacteria may settle at the site of a bone fracture and cause acute osteomyelitis.

Seventh Characters

Most categories in Chapter 19 require seventh characters that identify the encounter.

Most categories in this chapter have three seventh character values: A, initial encounter, D, subsequent encounter, and S, sequela. Categories for traumatic fractures have additional seventh character values.

The seventh character A is used while the patient is receiving active treatment for the condition. Examples of active treatment are surgical treatment, emergency department encounter, and evaluation and treatment by a new physician. The seventh character D is used for encounters after the patient has received active treatment of the condition and is receiving routine care for the condition during the healing or recovery phase. Examples of subsequent care are cast change or removal, removal of external or internal fixation device, medication adjustment, and other aftercare and follow-up visits following treatment of the injury or condition. The aftercare Z codes should not be used for aftercare for conditions such as injuries or poisonings, where seventh characters are provided to identify subsequent care.

Seventh character S is used for complications or conditions that arise as a direct result of a condition such as scar formation after a burn. The scars are sequelae of the burn. When using seventh character S, it is necessary to use both the injury code that precipitated the sequela and the code for the sequela itself. The S is added only to the injury code and not to the sequela code. The specific type of sequela is sequenced first, followed by the injury code.

When a subcategory code has less than six characters, a placeholder is used to maintain the position of the seventh character. For example, a closed fracture of the vault of the skull with subdural hemorrhage is reported with code S02.0XXA.

Main Terms for Injuries

The Alphabetic Index classifies injuries according to the general type of injury, such as a wound, fracture, or dislocation. The subterms under the general type of injury identify the anatomical site. For example:

> **Wound, open**
> > abdomen, abdominal
> > > wall, S31.109
> > > > with penetration into peritoneal cavity, S31.602
> > > ankle, S91.00-

Fractures

A break in a bone caused by traumatic injury or a disease process is known as a fracture. Fractures are coded by the bone involved and the nature of the break. To code fractures accurately and completely, the following questions must be answered:

- Is the fracture traumatic or pathologic? Review the health record for mention of trauma or underlying pathology, such as osteoporosis or bone metastasis. Pathological fractures are not considered traumatic and are not classified to Chapter 19 in the ICD-10-CM code book.

- Where is the fracture located? Review diagnostic studies, such as x-rays, to identify the specific location.
- Is the fracture open or closed?
- What is the laterality of the injury?

Closed fractures (with or without delayed healing) include the following terms:

Comminuted	Impacted
Depressed	Linear
Elevated	Simple
Fissured	Slipped epiphysis
Fracture, NOS	Spiral
Greenstick	

Open fractures (with or without delayed healing) are further described with the following terms:

Compound	Puncture
Infected	With foreign body
Missile	

A fracture not indicated as closed or open should be classified as closed. In the rare instance when a fracture is described as both open or closed, the code for Open is used. A fracture is described as displaced or not displaced in ICD-10-CM. The default code is to a displaced fracture.

Coders are permitted to use an x-ray report to assign a more specific fracture diagnosis code when the physician has documented a fracture. The physician may not list the specific site of the fracture, but an x-ray report in the health record shows the precise site. It is appropriate for the coder to assign the more specific code from the x-ray report without consulting the physician; however, when there is any question as to the appropriate diagnosis, the coder must contact the physician.

Category and subcategory codes include the following:

- S02   Fractures of skull and facial bones
- S12   Fractures of cervical vertebra and other parts of neck
- S22   Fractures of rib(s), sternum and thoracic spine
- S32   Fractures of lumbar spine and pelvis
- S42   Fractures of shoulder and upper arm
- S49.0–.1   Physeal fractures of shoulder and upper arm
- S52   Fracture of forearm
- S59.0–.1   Physeal fractures of elbow and forearm
- S62   Fracture of wrist and hand level
- S72   Fracture of femur
- S79.0–.1   Physeal fractures of hip and thigh
- S82   Fractures of lower leg, including ankle
- S89   Physeal fractures of lower leg
- S92.0–S92.3 Fracture of foot and toe, except ankle

Additional seventh characters are available to identify specific encounters for fracture coding. Seventh characters for fractures are unique to each type of bone and type of fracture. It is necessary to review the fracture seventh characters carefully before assigning a seventh character.

Fracture seventh characters are expanded to include the following:

A—Initial encounter for closed fracture
B—Initial encounter for open fracture
D—Subsequent encounter for fracture with routine healing
G—Subsequent encounter for fracture with delayed healing
K—Subsequent encounter for fracture with nonunion
P—Subsequent encounter for fracture with malunion
S—Sequela

Fracture categories provide for seventh characters to designate the specific type of open fracture (these designations are based on the Gustilo open fracture classification):

B—Initial encounter for open fracture type I or II (open not otherwise specified [NOS])
C—Initial encounter for open fracture type IIIA, IIIB, or IIIC
E—Subsequent encounter for open fracture type I or II with routine healing
F—Subsequent encounter for open fracture type IIIA, IIIB, or IIIC with routine healing
H—Subsequent encounter for open fracture type I or II with delayed healing
J—Subsequent encounter for open fracture type IIIA, IIIB, or IIIC with delayed healing
M—Subsequent encounter for open fracture type I or II with nonunion
N—Subsequent encounter for open fracture type IIIA, IIIB, or IIIC with nonunion
Q—Subsequent encounter for open fracture type I or II with malunion
R—Subsequent encounter for open fracture type IIIA, IIIB, or IIIC with malunion

Those fracture categories with distinct seventh characters include S02, S12, S22, S32, S42, S49, S52, S59, S62, S72, S79, S82, S89, and S92.

Fractures are not coded using the aftercare codes (Z codes). For encounters after the patient has completed active treatment of the fracture and is receiving routine care for the fracture during the healing or recovery phase, the fracture should be coded with the correct seventh character to identify the specific encounter. Examples of fracture care are cast change or removal, removal of external or internal fixation device, medication adjustment, and follow-up visits following fracture treatment. The appropriate seventh character is used to describe the encounter.

> **EXAMPLE:** Patient has a fractured lateral malleolus of the right fibula four weeks before.
> Patient is admitted to the outpatient unit to have the internal pins removed.
> S82.61XD

Some specific coding guidelines relating to fractures include the following:

- Fractures of the skull and other facial bones are reported with category S02. Fourth characters identify the area of the skull fractured, and fifth characters provide additional specificity.
- When intracranial injuries (S06-) or open wounds (S01-) accompany fractures, these additional codes are used to describe the injuries.
- Codes for intracranial injuries (S06-) have fourth and fifth characters that describe the type of injury (concussion, edema, contusion, focal brain injury, and so on) and sixth characters that indicate whether there was a loss of consciousness associated with the injury and, if so, the amount of time the patient was unconscious. These sixth characters are based not only on time but also whether the patient returned to a pre-existing level of consciousness or not.

EXAMPLE: Closed fracture of vault of the skull with subdural hemorrhage

Patient was unconscious for 12 hours before he died.

S02.0XXA

S06.5X7A

- Vertebral fractures are classified according to the part of the spine that is affected; that is, the cervical spine (S12.-), thoracic spine (S22.0-), or lumbar spine (S32.0).

- Fourth characters for cervical fractures indicate the specific vertebra involved; fifth and sixth characters identify the type of fracture, such as stable or displaced; for thoracic and lumbar fractures, the fifth characters indicate the specific vertebra involved; and sixth characters identify the type of fracture, such as wedge compression, stable burst, or unstable burst. Some examples include the following:

  ▸ S12.0   Fracture of first cervical vertebra
         S12.00   Unspecified fracture of first cervical vertebra
              S12.000   Unspecified displaced fracture of first cervical vertebra

  ▸ S22.0   Fracture of thoracic vertebra
         S22.01   Fracture of first thoracic vertebra
              S22.010   Wedge compression fracture of first thoracic vertebra

  ▸ S32.0   Fracture of lumbar vertebra
         S32.02   Fracture of second lumbar vertebra
              S32.021   Stable burst fracture of second lumbar vertebra

Additional codes from categories S14, S24, and S34 are used to classify associated spinal cord injuries:

  ▸ S14.121   Central cord syndrome at C1 level of cervical spinal cord
  ▸ S14.132   Anterior cord syndrome at C2 level of cervical spinal cord
  ▸ S24.133   Anterior cord syndrome at T7–T10 level of thoracic spinal cord
  ▸ S34.124   Incomplete lesion of L4 level of lumbar spinal cord

- Rib fractures are identified with codes S22.3- and S22.4-, depending on the number of ribs affected.

  ▸ S22.31   Fracture of one rib, right side
  ▸ S22.32   Fracture of one rib, left side
  ▸ S22.41   Multiple fractures of ribs, right side
  ▸ S22.43   Multiple fractures of ribs, bilateral

- There are several category codes used to describe fractures of the extremities. These include codes S42, S49, S52, S59, S62, S72, S79, S82, S89, and S92. Fourth characters generally indicate the general part of the bone affected, while fifth characters indicate specific sites. The sixth characters are used to report laterality and whether the fracture is displaced or nondisplaced. Some examples of codes include the following:

  ▸ S42   Fracture of shoulder and upper arm
         S42.0   Fracture of clavicle
              S42.00   Fracture of unspecified part of clavicle
                  S42.001 Fracture of unspecified part of right clavicle

  ▸ S52   Fracture of forearm
         S52.1   Fracture of upper end of radius
              S52.11   Torus fracture of upper end of radius
                  S52.112   Torus fracture of upper end of left radius

▶ S72   Fracture of femur
    S72.1   Pertrochanteric fracture
        S72.12   Fracture of lesser trochanter of femur
            S72.122   Displaced fracture of lesser trochanter of left femur

▶ S82   Fracture of lower leg, including ankle
    S82.2   Fracture of shaft of tibia
        S82.22   Transverse fracture of shaft of tibia
            S82.224   Nondisplaced transverse fracture of shaft of right tibia

▶ S92   Fracture of foot and toe, except ankle
    S92.1   Fracture of talus
        S92.12   Fracture of body of talus
            S92.123   Displaced fracture of body of unspecified talus

Remember that seventh characters are required for the following circumstances:

- If multiple fractures of the same bone occur at different sites of the bone, individual codes are used to code each of the fractures.

- Pelvic fractures are classified to category S32. The pelvis is comprised of a group of bones (ischium, ilium, pubis, sacrum, and coccyx) that form a circle that supports the spine. Any or all of these bones can be fractured. Fracture of the pelvic circle is considered very severe. Examples of pelvic fractures include the following:

▶ S32.51   Fracture of superior rim of pubis
    S32.511   Fracture of superior rim of right pubis
    S32.512   Fracture of superior rim of left pubis

▶ S32.61   Avulsion fracture of ischium
    S32.611   Displaced avulsion fracture of right ischium
    S32.612   Displaced avulsion fracture of left ischium
    S32.614   Nondisplaced avulsion fracture of right ischium
    S32.615   Nondisplaced avulsion fracture of left ischium

Dislocations

A dislocation is the displacement of a bone out of its joint. The most common joints affected are the fingers, thumb, and shoulder. Pain and swelling occur, as well as loss of use of the injured part. For healing, the dislocation can be reduced and immobilized with a cast. ICD-10-CM classifies dislocations or displacements to the following categories:

- S03   Dislocation and sprain of joints and ligaments of head
- S13   Dislocation and sprain of joints and ligaments of neck level
- S23   Dislocation and sprain of joints and ligaments of thorax
- S33   Dislocation and sprain of joints and ligaments of lumbar spine and pelvis
- S43   Dislocation and sprain of joints and ligaments of shoulder girdle
- S53   Dislocation and sprain of joints and ligaments of elbow
- S63   Dislocation and sprain of joints and ligaments at wrist and hand level
- S73   Dislocation and sprain of joint and ligaments of hip
- S83   Dislocation and sprain of joints and ligaments of knee
- S93   Dislocation and sprain of joints and ligaments at ankle, foot and toe level

Internal Injury of Chest, Abdomen, and Pelvis

Internal injuries of the thorax, abdomen, and pelvis are classified to categories S24–S27 and S34–S37. Examples of the types of injuries reported in these categories include the following:

- S25.0   Injury of thoracic aorta
- S25.2   Injury of superior vena cava
- S27.0   Traumatic pneumothorax
- S27.1   Traumatic hemothorax
- S27.2   Traumatic hemopneumothorax
- S27.32   Contusion of lung
- S34.0   Concussion and edema of lumbar and sacral spinal cord
- S35.0   Injury of abdominal aorta
- S36.020   Minor contusion of spleen
- S36.021   Major contusion of spleen
- S36.112   Contusion of liver
- S36.114   Minor laceration of liver
- S36.115   Moderate laceration of liver
- S36.41   Primary blast injury of small intestine
- S37.011   Minor contusion of right kidney
- S37.052   Moderate laceration of left kidney

Cerebral Concussion

A cerebral concussion is a transient loss of consciousness (less than 24 hours) after a traumatic head injury. Although no intracranial damage occurs, the patient may experience bradycardia, hypotension, and respiratory arrest for a few seconds, as well as retrograde and posttraumatic amnesia. The patient is put under 48-hour observation to check for the development of complications. A CT scan may be performed to rule out any intracranial injury. ICD-10-CM classifies concussion to category S06.0X, with sixth characters that identify the level of consciousness and the length of time that a patient has been unconscious.

> **EXAMPLE:**   S06.0X0   Concussion without loss of consciousness
>
>   S06.0X1   Concussion with loss of consciousness of 30 minutes or less
>
>   S06.0X2   Concussion with loss of consciousness from 31 to 59 minutes
>
>   S06.0X3   Concussion with loss of consciousness of 1 hour to 5 hours 59 minutes

Cerebral Contusion and Laceration

Often caused by a blow to the head, a cerebral contusion is a more severe injury than a concussion. It refers to a bruise of the brain with bleeding into brain tissue, but without disruption of brain continuity. The loss of consciousness that occurs often lasts longer than it does with a concussion. A laceration or fracture often accompanies the contusion. Any type of laceration of the brain results in some destruction of brain tissue and a subsequent scarring that may cause posttraumatic epilepsy. ICD-10-CM classifies cerebral contusion and laceration to category S06.3-, which further subdivides to identify the following:

- The specific part of the brain affected (brainstem, cerebrum, or cerebellum)
- The level of consciousness, as indicated by a sixth character

EXAMPLE: S06.31 Contusion and laceration of right cerebrum

S06.311 Contusion and laceration of right cerebrum with loss of consciousness of 30 minutes or less

S06.316 Contusion and laceration or right cerebrum with loss of consciousness greater than 24 hours without return to pre-existing conscious level with patient surviving

S06.37 Contusion, laceration, and hemorrhage of cerebellum

S06.371 Contusion, laceration and hemorrhage of cerebellum with loss of consciousness of 30 minutes or less

Sprains and Strains

A sprain is a stretching or tearing injury of the supporting ligaments of a joint, which results from the turning or twisting of a body part beyond its normal range of motion. Sprains are characterized by extreme pain, swelling, and discoloration, and they require rest for the injury to heal. Whiplash is a specific type of sprain constituting a compression of the cervical spine that involves the bones, joints, and intervertebral disks, usually due to a sudden throwing of the head forward and then backward.

A strain is a simple overstretching or overexertion of some part of a musculotendinous structure (muscle and tendon) that usually responds to rest. Patients may also suffer from chronic strains of the neck or back or derangements of different joints. The physician may describe these conditions as chronic, old, or recurrent. Using terms such as *sprain, strain* or *derangement*, the coder should refer to the subterm for the site and another subterm to describe the chronic, old, or recurrent condition. The coder will be referred to codes within the diseases of the musculoskeletal system categories (Chapter 13). The codes for sprains and strains are located within each block, depending on the anatomical site. Some examples include the following:

- S16.1   Strain of muscle, fascia and tendon at neck level
- S23.3   Sprain of ligaments of thoracic spine
- S43.5   Sprain of acromioclavicular joint
- S63.511 Sprain of carpal joint of right wrist
- S66.812 Strain of other specified muscles, fascia and tendons at wrist and hand level, left hand
- S93.512 Sprain of interphalangeal joint of left great toe

Open Wounds

An open wound is an injury of the soft tissue parts associated with rupture of the skin. Wounds may be described as crushed, incised, punctured, or penetrating, for example. A penetrating wound involves the passage of an object through tissue, leaving an entrance and exit wound, as in the case of a knife or gunshot wound. The seriousness of a wound depends on its site and extent. When a major vessel or organ is involved, a wound may be life threatening. For example, the rupture of a large artery or vein may cause blood to accumulate in one of the body cavities. This is referred to as hemothorax, hemopericardium, hemoperitoneum, or hemarthrosis, depending on the body cavity involved. The significance of the hemorrhage depends on the volume and rate of blood loss and the site of the hemorrhage. Large losses may induce hemorrhagic shock.

In ICD-10-CM, open wounds are classified to categories S01, S11, S21, S31, S41, S51, S61, S71, S81, and S91. The coder is reminded in each of these categories to code any associated injuries or wound infections. Some examples include the following:

- S11.011 Laceration without foreign body of larynx
- S11.024 Puncture wound with foreign body of trachea
- S21.132 Puncture wound without foreign body of left front wall of thorax without penetration into thoracic cavity
- S31.651 Open bite of abdominal wall, left upper quadrant with penetration into peritoneal cavity
- S41.021 Laceration with foreign body of right shoulder
- S51.822 Laceration with foreign body of left forearm
- S61.325 Laceration with foreign body of left ring finger with damage to nail
- S71.112 Laceration without foreign body, left thigh
- S81.041 Puncture wound with foreign body, right knee

Crushing Injuries

Crushing injuries quite often occur in the industrial setting. Avulsion (tearing away) of skin and fat or a friction burn of the tissues may result. Abrasion burns are often severe, including third degree. Vessels, nerves, and muscles may be avulsed, and bones may be dislocated or fractured. A common complication is secondary congestion, which can lead to paralysis and severe muscle fibrosis and joint stiffness. Often the overall circulation of the extremity is of greater concern than definitive management of specific structures. Some examples of codes for crush injuries include the following:

- S07.1   Crushing injury of skull
- S17.0   Crushing injury of larynx and trachea
- S57.01   Crushing injury of right elbow
- S87.02   Crushing injury of left knee
- S97.01   Crushing injury of right ankle
- S97.111 Crushing injury of right great toe

Traumatic Amputations

Traumatic amputations are classed as partial or complete. The default code is for the complete amputation. The term *amputation* is also used to describe the surgical procedure to remove part of a limb or an entire limb.

- S08.112 Complete traumatic amputation of left ear
- S28.211 Complete traumatic amputation of right breast
- S38.222 Partial traumatic amputation of penis

- S48.011   Complete traumatic amputation at right shoulder joint
- S58.122   Partial traumatic amputation at level between elbow and wrist, left arm
- S68.511   Complete traumatic transphalangeal amputation of right thumb
- S78.122   Partial traumatic amputation at level between left hip and knee

Burns

The ICD-10-CM makes a distinction between burns and corrosions. The burn codes are for thermal burns, except sunburns, that come from a heat source such as a fire or hot appliance. The burn codes are also for burns resulting from electricity and radiation. Corrosions are burns due to chemicals.

Current burns (T20–T25) are classified by depth, extent, and agent. By depth, burns are classified as first, second, and third degree. A first degree burn is the least severe and involves damage to the epidermis or outer layer of skin alone. A second degree burn involves the epidermis and dermis. There is edema and blistering of the skin, which is red and moist. A third degree burn is the most severe and includes all three layers of skin: epidermis, dermis, and subcutaneous. The skin appears charred, white, and dry.

Some examples of burn codes include the following:

- T20.1   Burn of first degree of head, face and neck

    T20.11   Burn of first degree of ear

    T20.111   Burn of first degree of right ear

    T20.112   Burn of first degree of left ear

- T20.2   Burn of second degree of head, face and neck

    T20.22   Burn of second degree of lip(s)

- T21.1   Burn of first degree of trunk

    T21.11   Burn of first degree of chest wall

    T21.14   Burn of first degree of lower back

- T22.2   Burn of second degree of shoulder and upper limb, except wrist and hand

    T22.23   Burn of second degree of upper arm

    T22.232   Burn of second degree of left upper arm

- T25.2   Burn of second degree of ankle and foot

    T25.23   Burn of second degree of toe(s)(nail)

    T25.232   Burn of second degree of left toe(s)(nail)

Burns of the eye and internal organs (T26–T28) are classified by site but not by degree. When a patient has both internal and external burns, the circumstances of admission govern the selection of the principal or first-listed diagnosis. When a patient is admitted for burn injuries and other related conditions, such as smoke inhalation or respiratory failure, the circumstances of admission govern the selection of the principal or first-listed diagnosis. Examples of codes from categories T26–T28 include the following:

- T26   Burn and corrosion confined to eye and adnexa

    T26.0   Burn of eyelid and periocular area

    T26.00   Burn of unspecified eyelid and periocular area

    T26.01   Burn of right eyelid and periocular area

    T26.02   Burn of left eyelid and periocular area

- T27   Burn and corrosion of respiratory tract

    T27.0   Burn of larynx and trachea

    T27.1   Burn involving larynx and trachea with lung

- T28   Burn and corrosion of other internal organs

    T28.0   Burn of mouth and pharynx

    T28.1   Burn of esophagus

    T28.2   Burn of other parts of alimentary tract

Categories T20–T28 must use the seventh character extension to identify the initial encounter (A), sequela (S), or subsequent encounter (D).

Codes from category T31, Burns classified according to extent of body surface involved, are assigned when the site of the burn is not specified or when there is a need for additional data. It is advisable to use category T31 as additional coding when needed to provide data for evaluating burn mortality, such as that needed by burn units. It is also advisable to use category T31 as an additional code for reporting purposes when there is mention of a third degree burn involving 20 percent or more of the body surface. Category T31 is based on the classic rule of nines in estimating body surface involved: head and neck are assigned 9 percent; each arm, 9 percent; each leg, 18 percent; anterior trunk, 18 percent; posterior trunk, 18 percent; and genitalia, 1 percent (see figure 19.1). Physicians may change these percentage assignments, when necessary, to accommodate infants and children who have proportionately larger heads than adults, as well as patients whose abdomens, buttocks, or thighs are proportionately larger than normal.

Current burns also are classified by depth, extent, and, where needed, agent. The following coding guidelines apply to burn injuries:

1. Code all burns with the highest degree of burn sequenced first.

2. Classify burns of the same local site but of different degrees, to the subcategory identifying the highest degree recorded in the diagnosis.

Figure 19.1.   Rule of nines

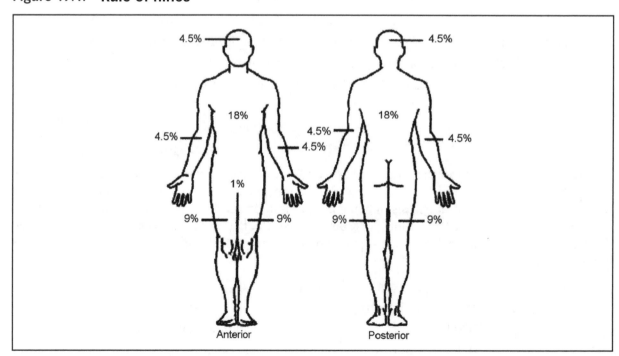

3. Code nonhealing burns as current acute burns. Code necrosis of burned skin as a nonhealed burn.

4. When a patient is admitted for burn injuries and other related conditions, such as smoke inhalation or respiratory failure, the circumstances of admission govern the selection of the principal or first-listed diagnosis.

Sunburn and other ultraviolet radiation burns are reported using codes from Chapter 12, Diseases of the skin and subcutaneous tissue. Sunburns can be described as first, second, or third degree burns.

Effects of Foreign Bodies Entering through Orifice

Foreign objects often are found in various body openings in the pediatric population. Children may insert small items into the nose or ear or swallow coins or marbles.

Foreign objects also may lodge in the larynx, bronchi, or esophagus, usually during eating. Laryngeal foreign bodies may produce hoarseness, coughing, and gagging, and partially obstruct the airway, causing stridor. Grasping forceps through a direct laryngoscope can remove laryngeal foreign bodies.

Bronchial foreign bodies usually produce an initial episode of coughing followed by an asymptomatic period, before obstructive and inflammatory symptoms occur. Bronchial foreign bodies are removed through a bronchoscope.

Esophageal foreign bodies produce immediate symptoms, such as difficulty in swallowing and coughing or gagging with the sensation of something stuck in the throat. These can be removed through an esophagoscope.

Intraocular foreign bodies require removal by an ophthalmic surgeon. Examples of foreign materials that can affect the eyes include airborne debris, metal fragments, and dislodged contact lenses.

ICD-10-CM classifies foreign bodies in orifices to various categories in Chapter 19. These categories are further subdivided to identify the specific site or orifice or whether the foreign body was accidentally left in following a proceduree. These codes can be found in the Alphabetic Index by referencing the main term *foreign body* and the subterm *entering through orifice*.

Some examples of codes relating to foreign bodies include the following:

- T15.00   Foreign body in cornea, unspecified eye
- T17.0   Foreign body in nasal sinus
- T17.22   Food in pharynx
- T18.0   Foreign body in mouth
- T18.4   Foreign body in colon
- T19.3   Foreign body in uterus

Injuries Resulting from Other and Unspecified Effects of External Causes

ICD-10-CM has codes to describe conditions that are the result of external causes, such as radiation sickness, frostbite, heatstroke or sunstroke, mountain sickness, and electric shock, as well as adverse effects not classified elsewhere. Specific categories are discussed in the following subsections.

Frostbite

Categories T33–T34 includes codes that describe conditions of reduced temperature:

- T33.011   Superficial frostbite of right ear
- T33.532   Superficial frostbite of left fingers
- T34.011   Frostbite with tissue necrosis of right ear
- T34.531   Frostbite with tissue necrosis of right fingers

Effects of Heat and Light

Category T67 includes codes that describe the effects of heat and light:

- T67.0   Heatstroke and sunstroke
- T67.1   Heat syncope
- T67.2   Heat cramp
- T67.3   Heat exhaustion, anhydrotic (due to water depletion)
- T67.4   Heat exhaustion due to salt depletion
- T67.5   Heat exhaustion, unspecified
- T67.6   Heat fatigue, transient
- T67.7   Heat edema
- T67.8   Other specified heat effects
- T67.9   Effect of heat and light, unspecified

Adverse Effects, Not Elsewhere Classified

Category T78 includes codes that describe adverse effects not classified elsewhere in ICD-10-CM. For example, anaphylactic reaction (T78.0) is a reaction marked by a sudden onset of rapidly progressing urticaria and respiratory distress. This code is appropriate in situations when anaphylactic shock is due to an adverse effect of a correct medicinal substance properly administered or to situations not otherwise specified. Underlying conditions should be coded first, such as poisonings by drugs, medicinals, and biologic substances chiefly nonmedicinal as to the source. Some examples of the codes in category T68 include the following:

- T78.01   Anaphylactic reaction due to peanuts
- T78.02   Anaphylactic reaction due to shellfish (crustaceans)
- T78.03   Anaphylactic reaction due to other fish
- T78.04   Anaphylactic reaction to fruits and vegetables
- T78.05   Anaphylactic reaction to tree nuts and seeds
- T78.06   Anaphylactic reaction due to food additives
- T78.07   Anaphylactic reaction due to milk and dairy products

Z Codes

There are several Z codes that are used to report aftercare for injuries. Patients with orthopedic injuries are likely to be seen in subsequent encounters for quite a long period of time following the initial injury.

Aftercare for fractures (for example, removal of pins, screws, or casts) are coded with the acute fracture coded with the appropriate seventh character value for subsequent care. Other types of non-fracture-related injuries that require aftercare will be reported with Z codes. Some examples include the following:

- Z47.1   Aftercare following joint replacement surgery
- Z47.2   Encounter for removal of internal fixation device
- Z47.31   Aftercare following explantation of shoulder joint prosthesis
- Z47.33   Aftercare following explantation of knee joint prosthesis
- Z47.82   Encounter for orthopedic aftercare following scoliosis surger

Z codes may also be used to identify an orthopedic status when it applies to an episode of care. For example, these status orders include the following:

- Z89.23   Acquired absence of shoulder
- Z89.5   Acquired absence of leg below knee
- Z96.611 Presence of right artificial shoulder joint
- Z97.13   Presence of artificial right leg (complete)(partial)
- Z98.1   Arthrodesis status

External Causes of Morbidity (V01–Y99)

External cause codes provide data for research on injuries and for evaluation of injury prevention strategies. These codes capture how the injury occurred, the intent, the place of occurrence, the activity of the patient at the time of the event, and the person's status. The beginning of Chapter 20, External cause of morbidity, offers a lot of information on the use of these codes and should be read very carefully. In addition, there are detailed notes at the beginning of blocks, category codes and subcategory codes.

General coding guidelines for external cause of morbidity codes include the following:

- These codes can be used with any code in the range of A00.0–T88.9, Z00–Z99
- External cause codes are used for each encounter in which the injury or condition is being treated.
- Use as many codes as necessary to fully explain the injury.
- External cause codes can never be a principal diagnosis code.

Some of the major categories of External Cause of Morbidity include the following:

V00–V99	Transport accidents
W00–X58	Other external causes of accidental injury
X71–X83	Intentional self-harm
X92–Y09	Assault
Y21–Y33	Event of undetermined intent
Y35–Y38	Legal intervention, operations of war, military operations, and terrorism
Y62–Y84	Complications of medical and surgical care
Y90–Y99	Supplementary factors related to causes of morbidity classified elsewhere

Place of Occurrence Guidelines

Codes from category Y92, Place of occurrence of the external cause, are secondary code for use after other external cause codes to identify the location of the patient at the time of injury or other condition. The place of occurrence code is used only one time at the initial encounter. A code from

Y92.9 is not used if the place is not stated. Some examples of place of occurrence codes include the following:

- Y92.01   Single-family non-institutional house as the place of occurrence of the external cause

    Y92.010   Kitchen of single-family house

    Y92.013   Bedroom of single-family house

- Y92.03   Apartment as the place of occurrence of the external cause

    Y92.031   Bathroom in apartment

- Y92.13   Military base as the place of occurrence of the external cause

    Y92.133   Barracks on military base

    Y92.137   Garden or yard

- Y92.23   Hospital as the place of occurrence of the external cause

    Y92.232   Corridor of hospital

    Y92.234   Operating room of hospital

- Y92.31   Athletic court as the place of occurrence of the external cause

    Y92.310   Basketball court as the place of occurrence

- Y92.82   Wilderness area

    Y92.820   Desert

Activity Code Guidelines

A code from Y93, Activity code, is used to describe the activity that the patient was engaged in at the time of the injury or other health condition. It is used only one time at the initial encounter for treatment. The activity codes are not applicable to poisonings, adverse effects, misadventures, or sequela. Do not assign code Y93.9, Unspecified activity, if the activity is not stated. Examples of activity codes include the following:

- Y93.0   Activities involving walking and running

    Y93.02   Activity, running

- Y93.2   Activities involving ice and snow

    Y93.21   Activity, ice skating

- Y93.3   Activities involving climbing, rappelling and jumping off

    Y93.32   Activity, rappelling

- Y93.D   Activities involving arts and handicrafts

    Y93.D2   Activity, sewing

- Y93.F   Activities involving caregiving

    Y93.F2   Activity, lifting

- Y93.K   Activities involving animal care

    Y93.K3   Activity, grooming and shearing an animal

External Cause Status Guidelines

A code from category Y99, External cause status, is assigned whenever any other external cause code is assigned for an encounter. It is used to indicate the work status of the person at the time the event occurred. For example, Y99.0 is used to report civilian activity done for income or pay.

Index to External Causes

The Index to External Causes is a separate index that follows the Table of Drugs and Chemicals (in most code books). It is organized by main terms (in boldface type) describing the accident, circumstance, event, or specific agent that caused the injury or other adverse effect, such as collision, earthquake, or dog bite, as in the following example:

Bite

    alligator W58.01

    bull W55.21

    cat W55.01

    dog W54.0

    goat W55.31

Coding Guidelines for External Cause Codes

The general guidelines related to the use of external cause codes include the following:

1. External cause codes for child and adult abuse take precedence over all other external cause codes.

2. External cause codes for terrorism events take precedence over all other external cause codes, except for child and adult abuse.

3. External cause codes for cataclysmic events take precedence over all other external cause codes, except for terrorism and child and adult abuse.

4. Transport accidents take precedence over all other external cause codes, except those for cataclysmic events, child and adult abuse, and terrorism.

5. Activity and external cause status codes are reported following other external cause code should correspond to the cause of the most serious diagnosis.

Terrorism Guidelines

When the cause of an injury is identified by the FBI as terrorism, the first-listed external cause code should be a code from category Y38, Terrorism. The definition of terrorism used by the FBI is found at the inclusion note at Y38.

Adult and Child Abuse, Neglect, and other Maltreatment, Ruled Out

If a suspected case of abuse, neglect, or mistreatment is ruled out during an encounter code, code T76, Adult and child abuse, neglect and other maltreatement, is not used. Instead, code Z04.71, Encounter for examination and observation following alleged physical adult abuse, ruled out, or code Z04.72, Encounter for examination and observation following alleged child physical abuse, ruled out, should be used. If a suspected case of alleged rape or sexual abuse is ruled out during an encounter code Z04.41, Encounter for examination and observation following alleged physical adult abuse, ruled out, or code Z04.42, Encounter for examination and observation following alleged rape or sexual abuse, ruled out, should be used. Again, a code from category T76 would not be used.

Poisonings, Toxic Effects, Adverse Effects, and Underdosing of Drugs

Conditions due to drugs and medicinal and biological substances are classified to categories T36–T50. These codes are combination codes that identify the responsible substance and whether it is a poisoning, an adverse effect, or an underdosing. If the condition is deemed a poisoning, the codes are further differentiated as to whether it was accidental, intentional self harm, an assault, or undetermined.

> **EXAMPLE:** T39.01   Poisoning by, adverse effect of, and underdosing of aspirin
>
>   T39.011   Poisoning by aspirin, accidental (unintentional)
>
>   T39.012   Poisoning by aspirin, intentional self-harm
>
>   T39.013   Poisoning by aspirin, assault
>
>   T39.014   Poisoning by aspirin, undetermined
>
>   T39.015   Adverse effect of aspirin
>
>   T39.016   Underdosing of aspirin

A special index called the Drug and Chemical Table follows the Alphabetic Index to Diseases and Injuries. It is used to code poisonings, adverse reactions, and underdosing.

The ICD-10-CM Table of Drugs and Chemicals is organized into seven columns with rows for the substances involved. The first, left-most column contains the name of the drug, chemical, or biologic substance. The next six columns contain the following:

- Poisoning, accidental (nonintentional)
- Poisoning, intentional self-harm
- Poisoning, assault
- Poisoning, undetermined
- Adverse effect
- Underdosing

Poisonings

Poisoning generally refers to conditions caused by drugs, medicinal substances, and other biological substances, when the substance involved is not used as prescribed. Poisonings can occur in the following manner:

- Overdose of medication given in error during a diagnostic or therapeutic procedure or during the course of medical care
- Overdose of medication given in error by nonmedical personnel, such as a mother to an infant or a child to an elderly parent
- Medication given to a wrong person by medical or nonmedical personnel
- Medication taken by wrong person
- Overdose of medication taken by self
- Intoxication (other than cumulative effect)
- Overdose
- Medications (prescription or nonprescription) taken in combination with alcoholic beverages
- Over-the-counter (OTC) medications taken in combination with prescribed medications without consulting a physician

When coding poisonings generally at least two codes are needed: one to report the poisoning and one to report the manifestation (tachycardia, delirium, gastrointestinal hemorrhaging, vomiting, hypokalemia, hepatitis, kidney failure, or respiratory failure, coma, tinnitus, rash, and so on). The poisoning code is sequenced as the principal diagnosis.

> **EXAMPLE:** Aspirin (over-the-counter pain medication) overdose resulting in a coma, intentional self-harm
>
> T39.012A and R40.20, Coma due to aspirin taken in a suicide attempt

> **EXAMPLE:** Lethargy due to accidental overdose of prescribed barbituates
>
> T42.3X1A and R53.83, Lethargy due to overdose of barbituates

When the poisoning is associated with abuse or dependence of the substance, the abuse or dependence is also coded.

Adverse Effects of Drugs

Adverse effects of, or reactions to, drugs can occur in situations where the medication is properly administered and correctly prescribed in both therapeutic and diagnostic procedures. Common causes of adverse effects include the following:

- Cumulative effects (often documented as drug toxicity in the health record) that result when the inactivation or excretion of the drug is slower than the rate at which the drug is being administered
- Hypersensitivities or allergic reactions that occur as qualitatively different responses to a drug, which are acquired only after re-exposure to the drug
- Synergistic reactions that enhance the effect of another drug administered prior to, or concurrent with, the drug
- Interactions with another prescribed medication that result in a change in the effectiveness of the drug
- Side effects that have unwanted, predictable pharmacologic effects that occur within therapeutic code ranges

> **EXAMPLE:** Atrial tachycardia due to digitalis glycosides toxicity. Patient took the medicine as prescribed
>
> I47.1 and T46.0X5A

> **EXAMPLE:** Premature supraventricular systole due to interaction between digitalis and Valium, both correctly prescribed and taken
>
> I49.3, T46.0X5A and T42.2X5A

Underdosing of Drugs

Underdosing refers to taking less of a medication than is prescribed by a provider or a manufacturer's instruction. For underdosing, assign the code from categories T36–T50 (fifth or sixth character). Codes for underdosing should never be assigned as principal or first-listed codes. If a patient has a relapse or exacerbation of the medical condition for which the drug is prescribed because of the reduction in dose, then the medical condition itself should be coded.

Noncompliance (Z91.12-, Z91.13-) or complication of care (Y63.61, Y63.8–Y63.9) codes are to be used with an underdosing code to indicate intent, if known.

Late Effects of Poisonings, Adverse Effects, and Underdosing of Drugs

When coding a late effect of a poisoning, the code for the substance is sequenced first (a code from T36–T50) with the seventh character for sequela (S). An additional code is used to identify the exact type of sequela. When coding a late effect of an adverse effect, assign a code for the manifestation or residual followed by a code from T36–T50 with the seventh character for sequela (S).

Seventh Characters

The seventh character for codes T36–T50 indicates whether the episode of care is the initial encounter (A), subsequent encounter (D), or sequela (S) of the past poisoning, adverse effect, or underdosing. An example of a combination code is T36.0X1A, Poisoning by penicillins, accidental (unintentional, initial encounter). No external cause of injury code is required to be added.

Toxic Effect of Nonmedicinal substances

T codes in ICD-10-CM are also available for coding the toxic effect of substances that are chiefly nonmedicinal in nature. For example, the code for toxic effect of carbon monoxide from motor vehicle exhaust, accidental (unintentional), initial encounter, is T58.01XA. Note that this is an example of a code that requires a seventh character but is less than six characters long (T58.01). In this code, a placeholder character of X is used to fill the missing sixth character. The seventh character must always be a valid seventh character in a code; it cannot take the place of a missing sixth character.

Chapter 19: ICD-10-CM Exercises

Review the following statements and cases and assign the appropriate codes:

1. Simple greenstick fracture, shafts of left tibia and fibula

2. Comminuted fracture of shaft of right femur

3. Fracture of right fibula due to osteogenesis imperfecta

4. Anterior dislocation of the left elbow

5. Chronic lumbosacral strain, subsequent encounter

6. Concussion without loss of consciousness

7. Laceration of left wrist, follow-up visit

8. Open frontal fracture with subarachnoid hemorrhage with loss of consciousness, less than 30 minutes

9. Cerebral contusion with loss of consciousness; patient regained consciousness on the second hospital day

10. Traumatic left below-the-knee amputation, follow-up visit

11. Spinal cord injury, C4 level, complete

12. First and second degree burns of the right palm

13. First degree burn of the left thigh and second degree burn of the left shoulder

14. Third degree burn of back involving 20 percent of body surface

15. Ataxia due to interaction of carbamazepine and erythromycin

16. Constipation from Oncovin injected for classical Hodgkin's disease

17. Hemiplegia resulting from previous adverse reaction to Enovid; left side of body. Patient is right-handed.

Assign diagnosis codes and external cause codes to the following statements and cases, as appropriate:

18. Fracture, right humerus (shaft); fell off ladder at home while cleaning gutters.

19. Intracapsular fracture, neck of left femur; patient slipped on ice and fell while playing hockey at school.

20. Fracture of second, third, and fourth ribs; patient was gored through the right chest by a bull. Patient is a bullfighter by profession and was gored by a bull while performing.

21. Chronic osteomyelitis of thigh due to an old compound fracture resulting from an automobile accident six months ago in which the patient was the driver

22. Scars of upper right arm due to an old grease burn sustained in a house fire three years ago

23. Inpatient admission: The patient is a 33-year-old construction worker who fell three stories from scaffolding at a construction site. He struck his head and was unconscious for about 10 minutes. An x-ray showed that he had an open parietal fracture with cerebral laceration and contusion. Patient complained of severe headache and dizziness.

    Discharge diagnoses: Headache and dizziness due to parietal bone fracture; cerebral laceration and contusions

24. Outpatient visit: The patient is a 10-year-old boy who had just returned from church camp. Apparently he ran into a raspberry patch while riding his bike and was punctured by thorns. This morning he awakened with a swollen, painful area on his left calf. On examination, the puncture wounds had healed and required no treatment, but the patient was prescribed antibiotics for cellulitis.

    Impression: Cellulitis due to *Streptococcus* group A

Continued

25. Inpatient admission: The patient was drinking heavily while at work in a movie theater when he slipped on the floor and dislocated his right shoulder. He is a known chronic alcoholic with cirrhosis of the liver. Laboratory tests were performed to monitor the status of the cirrhosis, and the shoulder was replaced to its proper position.

    Discharge diagnoses: Dislocated shoulder; alcoholic cirrhosis of the liver

26. Outpatient visit: A 31-year-old mine worker was severely burned several months ago while at work, when a propane tank exploded near his face. At the time, he had second- and third-degree burns of the face and neck. He was seen in consultation by a plastic surgeon for scarring of the skin. A grafting procedure was scheduled.

    Impression: Scarring of the face; late effect of second- and third-degree burns of the face and neck

27. Outpatient visit: The patient is a two-month-old girl who was seen for a severe rash all over the body. She had been given penicillin last week for bilateral suppurative otitis media. The physician examined her ears, which were still inflamed, and prescribed a sulfa drug for her ears and lotion for her rash.

    Impression: Severe rash due to penicillin; acute suppurative otitis media

28. Outpatient visit #1: The patient was seen by the physician with acute exacerbation of her asthma. The physician prescribed antibiotics, bronchodilators, and IV steroids.

    Impression: Acute exacerbation of asthma

    Outpatient visit #2: The patient was seen experiencing jitters and anxiety due to an accidental overdose of her bronchodilator that had been prescribed for her asthma, which is currently under control. She was cautioned to be careful about dosage amounts.

    Impression: Accidental overdose of Solu-Medrol; asthma

29. Emergency department visit: A 22-year-old female was brought to the emergency department in a semicomatose state. Her fiancé indicated that she drank between five and eight beers at dinner and then had taken Valium to sleep. She was unresponsive.

    Impression: Adverse reaction to alcohol and drugs

30. Inpatient admission: History of present illness: This 16-year-old boy was involved in a one-car accident at approximately 2 a.m. Apparently, the car skidded on some oil or water on the road and struck a mailbox on a residential street. The patient was an unrestrained passenger who either struck the windshield or was thrown through it. He was diagnosed with an L-1 fracture, neurologically intact. In addition, he was noted to have a laceration of his left frontal parietal area. The laceration was debrided and repaired.

    Pertinent lab and x-ray findings: WBC count on admission is 12.7; Hg and Hct 13.2 and 37.1, respectively; sodium 134; potassium 3.9; chloride 100; bicarb 25; glucose 96; creatinine 0.8; and BUN 7. Urinalysis also done on admission shows 3+ blood, 5 to 10 white cells, greater than 50 RBCs, otherwise unremarkable. Admission urine culture and sensitivity showed no growth. Blood flow studies showed the following impression: normal venous Doppler study. Thoracolumbar spine films showed the following: two views demonstrate a fracture of the first lumbar vertebral body. Most of the fracture involves the superior end plate. There is narrowing of the posterior aspect of the L-1/2 disk space, perhaps slight widening anteriorly. There are no other findings.

Pertinent physical findings: Patient is moving all extremities to command. He has no evidence of cyanosis or edema, and there are no palpable bony or joint abnormalities. He is drowsy but easily arousable. He is oriented times three. He responds appropriately to questions when asked. His sensation is intact to touch and pinprick throughout. Lower extremities 5/5 in all groups bilaterally. Deep tendon reflexes 2+ and equal bilaterally.

Hospital course: The patient was admitted to assess neurologic integrity and to begin definitive rehabilitation. As previously mentioned, although suffering from an L-1 fracture, the patient was neurologically intact. He was treated symptomatically for pain discomfort and to protect the spine. Then, he was fitted with a lumbosacral orthosis and began sitting gradually. The patient tolerated that well and was ready for discharge. He was discharged home in the care of his mother with a prescription for the following medication: Vicodin, 1 po q-4h prn for pain. At discharge, he was medically stable and on a regular diet. The patient was instructed to keep the brace on at all times, except when bathing. He was further instructed to log roll when in bed and not to stretch, bend, or twist back. The patient was told to walk as much as possible, wear tennis shoes when walking, and, when riding in the car, to wear the seat belt. If he experienced any numbness, tingling, or loss of sensation at any time, he was instructed to call his attending physician immediately.

Discharge diagnoses: Lumbar fracture from motor vehicle accident; no loss of consciousness; laceration of left frontal parietal area

Do not code external cause codes for the following questions:

31. A nine-month-old baby girl is brought to the doctor by her parents, who had observed her being shaken violently by the babysitter on a nanny cam. The physician diagnoses shaken baby syndrome and admits the baby to the hospital immediately.

32. Patient is seen with a skull fracture at the base of the skull. MRI shows a subarachnoid hemorrhage. There was a period of unconsciousness for up to 50 minutes.

33. The mother of a two-year-old brings the child to the physician's office after seeing him eat five tramadol from an opened medicine bottle.

34. Follow-up visit for a patient who had a trimalleolar fracture of the right ankle subsequent to a fall down a flight of steps. The x-ray showed a normally healing bone.

35. This patient is seen in the hospital with a diagnosis of congestive heart failure due to hypertensive heart disease. Patient also has stage V chronic kidney failure. The patient had been prescribed Lasix previously but admits that he forgets to take his medication every day. This is due to his advanced age. What are the correct diagnosis codes?

36. This former athlete is seen for increased left hip pain. He has a left hip prosthesis following an injury while playing professional football. A MRI shows an infection of the prosthesis.

37. A homeless man is admitted for an apparent suicide attempt with an overdose of marijuana and cocaine. While attempting to get to a nearby shelter, he fell and suffered a laceration of the left cheek and scalp. He is seen by the ED physician and stabilized.

38. The patient is a 22-year-old patient with deep third-degree burns of the chest and the right leg. He was involved in a house fire. He has third-degree burns over 22 percent of his body.

Continued

39. The young worker was crushed by a metal rolling mill machine at work. He was treated for crushing injuries to the left toes, foot, and right ankle.

40. The patient is a five-year-old girl who swallowed Drano at the age of three. She suffered acid burns to the mouth, throat, trachea, and esophagus and now presents with scarring to the esophagus and trachea. Plastic surgery will be attempted to remove scar tissue.

41. The patient is seen in the emergency department following a suicide attempt using barbiturates and acetaminophen. The patient is stable medically, underwent stomach lavage, and was transferred to the psychiatric unit for treatment of depression.

42. Stab wound to the abdominal wall with infection

43. Traumatic amputation of right arm above the elbow

44. Patient was seen with uncontrolled hypertension. He is elderly and on a fixed income and can't afford his hypertension medicine.

45. Patient is seen with hives and a dry mouth due to taking prescribed phenobarbital for anxiety.

46. Bradycardia in a three-year-old due to accidental ingestion of oleander leaves

Assign the external cause codes only for the following questions:

47. A college student driving her car collided with a truck on the highway. She was talking to her mother on the phone while driving.

48. A United States army major stationed on an international military base was struck by shrapnel after an IED explosion.

49. A postman was bitten by a stray dog while walking toward his postal truck in the parking lot of the post office.

50. A school cook was burned with hot oil while preparing lunch for the kindergarten school children.

Assign all diagnosis and external cause codes (including place of occurrence, activity, and external status codes) for the following questions:

51. This 60-year-old homeowner was changing shutters on his townhouse and fell from the ladder into the yard. He had a nondisplaced right radial fracture at the distal end. A cast was applied, and the patient was discharged. What diagnosis and external cause codes are assigned?

52. A patient fell from a ladder in the garage several weeks ago while working on a defective light fixture in the garage. The injury resulted in a fracture of L1 and L2 vertebral bodies. He is receiving massage therapy for this injury, and it is healing well. What diagnosis and external cause codes are assigned?

53. This 33-year-old was burned on her right shoulder by scalding water in her kitchen one week ago. She was treated and released and is now seen by the physician for a dressing change to her right shoulder. The burns were first- and second-degree burns to the shoulder.

54. This 19-year-old male was a driver involved in an automobile accident when he rear-ended another car on the highway. He was seen in the emergency department with severe pain in the lower right arm. He was treated for a displaced, open fracture type III of the shaft of the right radius and ulna. What diagnosis and external cause codes are assigned?

55. This eight-year-old is seen for follow-up of his elbow fracture. Eight weeks ago, this patient injured his elbow when he fell while playing basketball at the local recreation center. He collided with another player on the court. After further evaluation, the attending physician found a nonunion of the previously displaced left distal humerus fracture. What diagnosis and external codes are assigned?

56. This 28-year-old female was seen for an infection due to a laceration on the sole of her left foot. She had taken her shoes off at the time of the accident. This laceration occurred five days ago, but the patient didn't want to see the doctor; however, it became very painful. The patient reports that her foot was cut by broken glass at a local café, where she was visiting with friends. The patient admits that she is a chronic alcohol abuser. Antibiotics are given for the infection. The doctor removed a small segment of glass that was still in the wound. What diagnosis and external cause codes are assigned?

57. This patient is a 22-year-old college student who is brought to the emergency department by ambulance and found to be the victim of a brutal fight at a sports stadium following a championship game. The patient was comatose when found by the police. The paramedics documented a score of 14 on the Glasgow coma scale. The patient was in a coma on the scene but regained consciousness within 10 minutes of arriving in the ED. It is estimated that he was unconscious for at least 90 minutes. The MRI is negative for fractures or internal bleeding. The physician describes the injury as a closed head injury. What diagnosis and external cause codes are assigned?

58. This is an 88-year-old female who fell down the icy front steps of her apartment complex and sustained a nondisplaced closed fracture of the tibia of her left leg. Because of the possibility of head injury, a CT scan was done, which revealed a small subdural hematoma. The neurologist felt that the hematoma currently did not require any intervention. What diagnosis and external cause codes are assigned?

59. Fracture of the ulna due to a fall from a motorcycle while alighting in a parking lot. The patient was a passenger on the back of the motorcycle, initial encounter.

60. Laceration of the pinna of the right ear from an accidental human bite. The wound is infected.

61. A patient lacerated her big toe while cleaning her kitchen. She accidentally bumped her right foot on the cabinet. She is an unemployed homemaker, initial encounter.

Complications of Surgical and Medical Care

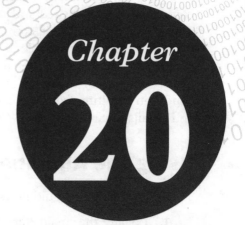

OBJECTIVES

After completing this lesson, you should be able to do the following:

- Apply knowledge of current, approved ICD-10-CM coding guidelines to assign and sequence accurate codes for diagnoses related to complications of surgical and medical care

- Identify locations in the Alphabetic Index, where terms relating to complications of surgical and medical care can be found

- Differentiate between mechanical complications and reactions of the body to foreign bodies such as grafts, implants, and other prosthetic devices

ICD-10-CM

Categories T80 through T88 are provided for complications of medical and surgical care not elsewhere classified. Like other categories in Chapter 19, categories T80–T85 and T88 require a seventh character to indicate either the initial encounter for treatment (A), the subsequent encounter (D), or the sequela (S) of care. Not all conditions that occur postoperatively are considered complications; they may be expected consequences of the surgery. Postoperative pain, nausea and vomiting, and anemia are rarely considered to be complications of surgery. Clear documentation must be provided by the physician to warrant the use of a complication code. When it is not clear whether there is a cause and effect relationship between the surgery and the condition, it is necessary to query the physician.

How to Determine Complications of Surgical or Medical Care

To properly classify complications, the coder must be certain that the complicating condition resulted from, or was caused by, the surgical or medical care rendered.

A time limit has not been designated for using categories T80–T88, because some complications may occur during or directly following surgery, during the same hospitalization, or several days, weeks, or months later.

In some cases, the documentation in the health record will clearly state a complication, such as colitis due to radiation therapy. In other cases, it will identify symptoms that may refer to a complication, such as red and warm surgical wound with drainage. Again, the physician should be asked to clarify whether a complication is present.

The note under the block title, Complications of surgical and medical care, not elsewhere classified, reminds the coder to "use additional code for adverse effect, if applicable, to identify drug" (T36–T50) with fifth or sixth character S, "use additional code(s) to identify the specified condition resulting from the complication," and "use additional code to identify devices involved and details of circumstances" (Y62–Y82).

Using the Alphabetic Index

The following coding guidelines apply to complications of surgical or medical care:

1. Locate the main term for the complication in the Alphabetic Index (for example, Malabsorption).

2. Check for a subterm indicating that the condition is a result of a complication of medical or surgical care, such as in the following example:

Malabsorption K90.9
postsurgical K91.2

---

3. If a specific code is not identified, look under Complications to locate an appropriate code by condition or system, such as in the following example:

Complications
    coronary aretery (bypass) graft T82.9
    electronic stimulator device
        bone T84.9
            breakdown T84.310
            displacement T84.320
        brain T85.9
            embolism T85.81
            fibrosis T85.82
            hemorrhage T85.83
    endocrine E34.9
        postprocedural
            adrenal hypofunction E89.6
            hypoinsulinemia E89.1
    esophagostomy K94.30
        hemorrhage K94.31
    genitourinary
        device or implant T83.9
            genital tract T83.9
                specified type NEC T83.89
                embolism T83.81

---

graft (bypass)(patch)
    bone T86.839
        failure T86.831
        infection T86.832
implant
    urinary sphincter T83.9
        embolism T83.81
        pain T83.84
intraoperative (intraprocedural)
    cardiac arrest
        during cardiac surgery I97.710
        during other surgery I97.711
    hemorrhage (hematoma)
        digestive system organ
            during procedure on digestive system K91.61
            during procedure on other organ K91.62
        puncture or laceration (accidental) (unintentional) (of)
        brain
            during a nervous system procedure G97.48
joint prosthesis, internal T84.9
    breakage (fracture) T84.01-
    dislocation T84.02-
    instability T84.02-
orthopedic
    device or implant
        breakdown T84.418
        fibrosis T84.82
        hemorrhage T84.83
        malposition T84.428
        obstruction T84.498
perfusion NEC T80.90
phototherapy T88.9
prosthetic device
    skin graft T86.829
        artificial skin or decellularized allodermis
            embolism T85.81
            infection and inflammation T85.79
            mechanical
                breakdown T85.613
                perforation T85.693
puncture, spinal G97.1
radiation
    kyphosis M96.2
    scoliosis M96.5
respirator
    mechanical J95.850

```
                stent
                    urinary T83.9
                        embolism T83.81
                        fibrosis T83.82
                        hemorrhage T83.83
                surgical procedure (on) T81.9
                    genitourinary NEC N99.89
                    hepatic failure K91.82
                    hyperglycemia E89.1
                    ovarian failure E89.40
                    postmastectomy lymphedema syndrome I97.2
                    shock (hypovolemic) T81.19
                    suture, permanent (wire) T85.9
                    tracheostomy J95.00
                transplant T86.90
                    bone T86.839
                        failure T86.831
                        rejection T86.830
                    heart T86.20
                        with lung T86.30
                vaccination T88.1
                    anaphylaxis NEC T80.52
                    cellulitis T88.0
                    encephalitis or encephalomyelitis G04.02
                    protein sickness T80.62
```

4. When the appropriate code cannot be found, assign the following nonspecific complication codes only when documentation in the health record supports their assignment:

Complications
    medical procedures T88.9
    surgical procedures T81.9

Complications Described as Postoperative Conditions

Often physicians describe a condition that arises after surgery as being postoperative, even though it is not a complication of the surgery. Coders should ask the attending physician for clarification when there is no causal relationship between the postoperative condition and the surgical procedure. For example, a patient's blood pressure dropped to 87/42 postoperatively in the recovery room following repair of a right, recurrent inguinal hernia. The attending physician ordered atropine 0.5 mg IV at 10:56 a.m. and again at 11:03 a.m. This episode of hypotension was not considered a complication of surgical care but rather a postoperative event.

Further, the attending physician should be queried about conditions such as postoperative fever and postoperative atelectasis (collapse of the lung) to determine whether these are expected occurrences from surgery or unexpected complications of surgical care. For example, an open-heart surgery patient's postoperative chest x-rays may show discoid atelectasis in both posterobasilar segments of the lung without evidence of pneumonia, edema, or failure. The physician should be queried as to whether the atelectasis was expected or unexpected and whether it required additional treatment (such as chest pulmonary toiletry or medication).

Postoperative anemia is actually rarely considered a complication of surgery. When the physician documents in the record that the patient has postoperative anemia due to blood loss, code D62, Acute posthemorrhagic anemia, is reported. This is not a complication code. The use of blood transfusions during or after surgery does not indicate that the anemia is a complication of surgery.

Complications Affecting Specific Body Systems

ICD-10-CM classifies many intraoperative and postoperative complications within the body system chapters, with codes specific to the organs of that body system. These codes are sequenced first, followed by codes for the specific complication. Some examples include the following:

- E89.0 Postprocedural hypothyroidism
- E89.1 Postprocedural hypoinsulinemia
- E89.3 Postprocedural hypopituitarism
- E89.40 Asymptomatic postprocedural ovarian failure
- G97.0 Cerebrospinal leak from spinal puncture
- G97.1 Other reaction to spinal and lumbar puncture
- G97.2 Intracranial hypotension following ventricular shunting
- G97.3 Intraoperative hemorrhage and hematoma of a nervous system organ structure complicating a procedure

  G97.31 Intraoperative hemorrhage and hematoma of a nervous system organ or structure complicating a nervous system procedure

  G97.32 Intraoperative hemorrhage and hematoma of a nervous system organ or structure complicating other procedure

- J95.0 Tracheostomy complications

  J95.00 Unspecified tracheostomy complication

  J95.01 Hemorrhage from tracheostomy stoma

  J95.02 Infection of tracheostomy stoma

- J95.1 Acute pulmonary insufficiency following thoracic surgery
- M96.1 Postlaminectomy syndrome, NEC

Complications Following Infusion, Transfusion, and Therapeutic Injections

Category T80 includes complications related to infusion, transfusion, or therapeutic injections. Some examples include the following:

- T80.0 Air embolism following infusion, transfusion and therapeutic injection
- T80.1 Vascular complication following infusion, transfusion and therapeutic injection
- T80.2- Infections following infusion, transfusion, and therapeutic injection

  T80.21 Infection due to central venous catheter

  T80.211 Bloodstream infection due to central venous catheter

T80.212   Local infection due to central venous catheter

T80.218   Other infection due to central venous catheter

- T80.3   ABO incompatibility reaction due to transfusion of blood or blood products

  T80.30   ABO incompatibility reaction due to transfusion of blood or blood products, unspecified

  T80.31   ABO incompatibility with hemolytic transfusion reaction

  T80.310   ABO incompatibility with acute hemolytic transfusion reaction

  T80.311   ABO incompatibility with delayed hemolytic transfusion reaction

- T80.4-   Rh incompatibility reaction due to transfusion of blood or blood products
- T80.5-   Anaphylactic shock due to serum
- T80.6-   Other serum reactions
- T80.81   Extravasation of vesicant agents
- T80.89   Other complications
- T80.9   Unspecified complications

Code T80.81- is used to report extravasation of agents, which is the accidental infiltration of intravenously infused drugs into the surrounding healthy tissue. Vesicants will cause blistering on the affected tissue. More seriously, extravasation of chemotherapy drugs may lead to serious complications, such as tissue necrosis or loss of limbs.

Complications Due to Presence of Internal Device, Implant, or Graft

Categories T82 through T85 are used to report conditions that occur because of internal devices, implants, or grafts. These complications are classified according to the body system involved:

- T82   Complications of cardiac and vascular prosthetic devices, implants and grafts
- T83   Complications of genitourinary prosthetic devices, implants and grafts
- T84   Complications of internal orthopedic prosthetic devices, implants and grafts
- T85   Complications of other internal prosthetic devices, implants and grafts

There are mechanical complications and nonmechanical complications. Mechanical complications include breakdown, displacement, leakage, or other malfunction. Some examples of mechanical complications include the following:

- T83.39-   Perforation of uterus by intrauterine contraceptive device
- T82.49-   Obstruction of arteriovenous dialysis catheter
- T84.01   Broken internal joint prosthesis
- T84.04   Periprosthetic fracture around internal prosthetic joint
- T84.01   Broken internal joint prosthesis
- T84.02   Dislocation of internal joint prosthesis
- T84.03   Mechanical loosening

Some examples of nonmechanical complications include the following:

- T82.6   Infection and inflammatory reaction due to cardiac valve prosthesis

- T82.7   Infection and inflammatory reaction due to other cardiac and vascular devices, implants and grafts
- T83   Complications of genitourinary prosthetic devices, implants and grafts
- T83.5   Infection and inflammatory reaction due to prosthetic device, implant and graft in urinary system
    - T83.51   Infection and inflammatory reaction due to indwelling urinary catheter
    - T83.59   Infection and inflammatory reaction due to prosthetic device, implant and graft in urinary system
- T83.6-   Infection and inflammatory reaction due to prosthetic device, implant, or graft in the genital tract
- T84.5-   Infection and inflammatory reaction due to internal joint prosthesis
    - T84.50   Infection and inflammatory reaction due to unspecified internal joint prosthesis
    - T84.51   Infection and inflammatory reaction due to internal right hip prosthesis
    - T84.52   Infection and inflammatory reaction due to internal left hip prosthesis
- T84.6-   Infection and inflammatory reaction due to internal fixation device
    - T84.61   Infection and inflammatory reaction due to internal fixation device of arm
        - T84.610   Infection and inflammatory reaction due to internal fixation device of right humerus
- T85.7-   Infection and inflammatory reaction due to other internal prosthetic devices, implants and grafts
    - T85.71   Infection and inflammatory reaction due to peritoneal dialysis catheter
    - T85.72   Infection and inflammatory reaction due to insulin pump
- T85.8-   Other specified complications of internal prosthetic devices, implants and grafts, NEC
    - T85.81   Embolism due to internal prosthetic devices, implants and grafts, NEC
    - T85.82   Fibrosis due to internal prosthetic devices, implants and grafts, NEC
- T85.9   Unspecified complication of internal prosthetic device, implant and graft

Transplant Complications

Codes describing complications of transplanted organs and tissue are found in Category T86. Code categories in T86 include the following:

- T86.0   Complications of bone marrow transplant
- T86.1   Complications of kidney transplant
- T86.2   Complications of heart transplant
- T86.3   Complications of heart-lung transplant
- T86.4   Complications of liver transplant
- T86.5   Complications of stem cell transplant
- T86.8   Complications of other transplanted organs and tissues
- T86.9   Complication of unspecified transplanted organ and tissue

Subcategory codes identify whether the complication is rejection, failure, or infection. Examples include:

- T86.01   Bone marrow transplant rejection
- T86.02   Bone marrow transplant failure
- T86.03   Bone marrow transplant infection
- T86.09   Other complications of bone marrow transplant

Subcategory code T86.8 is further subdivided into:

- T86.81   Complications of lung transplant
- T86.82   Complications of skin graft (allograft) (autograft)
- T86.83   Complications of bone graft
- T86.84   Complications of corneal transplant
- T86.85   Complication of intestine transplant
- T86.89   Complications of other transplanted tissue

Patients who have chronic kidney disease (CKD) following a transplant are not assumed to have transplant rejection or failure, unless the physician documents it as so. Patients may still have CKD if kidney function is not fully restored. Only a physician can make that determination.

When there is an accompanying infection, the coder is reminded to use an additional code from category B95 through B97. Generally two codes are required to fully describe a transplant complication: one is a code from category T86, and the other is the specific complication.

> **EXAMPLE:**   Acute graft versus host disease resulting from complication of bone marrow transplant
>
> T86.09 and D89.810

> **EXAMPLE:**   *Staphylococcal aureus* infection in transplanted kidney
>
> T86.13 and B95.61

Complications of Reattached Limbs and Amputations

Complications of reattached extremities and amputated stump are classified to category T87. Complications relating to reattached limbs are further specified by upper or lower limbs and then laterality. Phantom limb syndrome is reported with codes G54.6 and G54.7, depending on the presence or absence of pain. Some examples of codes include the following:

- T87.0   Complications of reattached (part of) upper extremity

    T87.0X   Complications of reattached (part of) upper extremity

    T87.0X1   Complications of reattached (part of) right upper extremity

    T87.0X2   Complications of reattached (part of) left upper extremity

    T87.0X9   Complications of reattached (part of) unspecified upper extremity

- T87.1   Complications of reattached (part of) lower extremity
- T87.2   Complications of other reattached body part
- T87.3   Neuroma of amputation stump
- T87.4   Infection of amputation stump
- T87.5   Necrosis of amputation stump

- T87.8   Other complication of amputation stump
- T87.9   Unspecified complications of amputation stump

Surgical or Medical Care as External Cause

ICD-10-CM provides external cause codes to indicate medical or surgical care as the cause of a complication. These codes include the following:

- Y62–Y69   Misadventures to patients during medical or surgical care
- Y70–Y82   Medical devices associated with adverse incidents in diagnostic and therapeutic care
- Y83–Y84   Surgical and other medical procedures as the cause of abnormal reaction of the patient, or later complication, without mention of misadventure at the time of the procedure

Codes Y62–Y69 are used when a condition is stated to be caused by some sort of misadventure during medical or surgical care. Some examples include the following:

- Y62.1   Failure of sterile precautions during infusion or transfusion
- Y63.0   Excessive amount of blood or other fluid given during a transfusion or infusion
- Y63.1   Incorrect dilution of fluid used during infusion
- Y64.0   Contaminated medical or biological substance, transfused or infused
- Y65.0   Mismatched blood in transfusion
- Y65.2   Failure in suture or ligature during surgical operation
- Y65.5   Performance of wrong procedure

   Y65.51   Performance of wrong procedure on correct patient

   Y65.53   Performance of correct procedure on wrong side or body part

Categories Y70–Y82 includes breakdown or malfunctions of medical devices. The subcategory codes include the following:

- Y70   Anesthesiology devices associated with adverse incidents
- Y71   Cardiovascular devices associated with adverse incidents
- Y72   Otorhinoloaryngological devices associated with adverse incidents
- Y73   Gastroenterology and urology devices associated with adverse incidents
- Y74   General hospital and personal use devices associated with adverse incidents
- Y75   Neurological devices associated with adverse incidents
- Y76   Obstetric and gynecological devices associated with adverse incidents
- Y77   Ophthalmic devices associated with adverse incidents
- Y78   Radiological devices associated with adverse incidents
- Y79   Orthopedic devices associated with adverse incidents
- Y80   Physical medicine devices associated with adverse incidents
- Y81   General and plastic surgery devices associated with adverse incidents
- Y82   Other and unspecified medical devices associated with adverse incidents

Codes from categories Y83 and Y84 are used when a condition is described as due to medical or surgical care but without mention of misadventure.

Chapter 20: ICD-10-CM Exercises

Review the following statements and cases and assign the appropriate codes:

1. Postoperative cellulitis of lower leg

2. Complication of breast implant

3. Infection of colostomy

4. Displacement of intrauterine contraceptive device

5. Urinary retention due to surgery

6. Air embolism due to intravenous infusion

7. Office visit: The patient was seen with persistent knee pain subsequent to insertion of a right knee prosthesis one year ago. X-ray revealed periprosthetic fracture around prosthetic joint. A recurrent thrombophlebitis was also noted in the right lower extremity, and Coumadin was ordered. The physician ordered physical therapy and antibiotics for the thrombophlebitis. The patient was scheduled for a right knee debridement and revision.

   Impression: Malfunctioning knee prosthesis; thrombophlebitis of right lower leg

   Code(s):

8. Office visit: The patient was seen for complaints of shortness of breath and productive cough. The physician ordered an injection of penicillin. The patient went into anaphylactic shock with acute respiratory failure. CPR was administered, and the patient was transported by ambulance to the emergency department.

   Impression: Upper respiratory infection; anaphylactic shock due to penicillin

9. Inpatient admission: The patient was admitted to the hospital for treatment of a cervical carcinoma. During the hysterectomy procedure, the patient had a cardiac arrest. The patient was resuscitated, and the operation continued. Prior to discharge, the patient developed a postoperative wound infection that was drained; IV antibiotics were started. Following aggressive treatment, the patient was discharged.

   Discharge diagnoses: Carcinoma of cervix; cardiac arrest during surgery; postoperative wound infection

10. Inpatient admission: A 50-year-old man was admitted with severe internal penile prosthesis infection and purulent drainage at the base of the left corpora. He has an 11-year history of type II diabetes mellitus. Blood glucose on admission was 160. The patient was admitted with a temperature of 99.2°F and a blood pressure of 138/88.

    Pertinent laboratory results:

    Blood glucose (normal values 65 to 110)

    12/28   122
    12/28   145
    12/28   128

12/28   140

12/31   134

01/01   162

01/08   152

01/11   130

Hct and Hb:

Normal values:

Hb: 13.5 to 18 male; 12 to 16 female

Hct: 40% to 54% male; 36% to 46% female

12/27   10.5/30.6

12/28   8.0/23.4

1/11   8.6/25.9

Urinalysis

12/27   WBC = 5–10

Blood = small

Sp. Gr. = 1.030

RBC = 1–5

C&S = Beta-hemolytic group B streptococcus; colony count >10,000

Hospital course: On 12/28, and after 24 hours of hydration, the patient was taken to the OR, where removal of an inflatable penile prosthesis was performed. The patient tolerated the procedure well and was taken to recovery in good condition. The patient received two weeks of oral antibiotics and was discharged on 1/12. Discharge medications were Cipro 500 mg po bid and Tylenol #3. The patient was discharged with an Accu-check machine to monitor his blood glucose levels, which were uncontrolled during the hospitalization, even with increased dosages of insulin. The patient's glucose levels will be checked daily on an outpatient basis to try to bring the levels into better control.

Discharge diagnoses: Infection of internal penile prosthesis due to group B *Streptococcus*; type II diabetes mellitus

11. Postprocedural hypertension

12. Severe headache due to lumbar puncture

13. Displaced lens implant in left eye

14. Erosion of skin of the chest wall due to pacemaker electrodes

15. Broken left hip prosthesis

16. The patient was in the Cardiac Cath Lab for insertion of a dual chamber pacemaker to treat his sick sinus syndrome. During the procedure the pacemaker electrode broke upon insertion. The procedure was abandoned and will be rescheduled. (Do not assign external cause codes.)

17. Postoperative pelvic adhesions

Continued

18. Subsequent encounter for a hematoma of a transabdominal myocutaneous (TRAM) flap following reconstruction of breast

19. Bone marrow transplant rejection syndrome; acute graft-versus-host disease

20. Postoperative cardiac arrest in the operating room during heart surgery

21. Hypovolemic post-op shock

22. MSSA infection of a transplanted kidney

23. Aspiration pneumonia following surgery

24. Infected pacemaker pocket due to *Streptococcus*, initial encounter

25. The patient is seen in the ED with abscess of the stump following a right below the knee amputation (BKA) six weeks ago. Patient has diabetes with peripheral angiopathy.

26. Persistent vomiting following gastrointestinal surgery one day ago

27. Phantom limb pain following amputation

28. The patient is a six-year-old female admitted to the hospital with shortness of breath and lethargy. The patient was seen last week to have an infusion catheter placed for initial administration of chemotherapy. Patient has acute lymphoblastic leukemia. X-rays show that the tip of the infusion catheter was broken off and positioned in the pulmonary artery.

29. The patient is a 32-year-old female who was discharged two days prior to this admission. She had a hysterectomy and was now experiencing severe dysuria, fever, and chills. The ED doctor noted that the incision site was red and extremely tender. Wound cultures grew *Staphylococcus aureus*. Urinalysis revealed *Escherichia coli*. The patient was started on antibiotics, and the symptoms abated within a few hours. The physician documents that the problems were postoperative complications of the hysterectomy. The final diagnoses included postoperative urinary tract infection and postoperative wound infection.

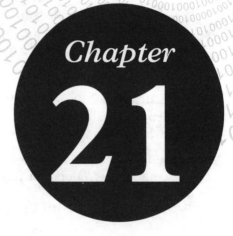

Factors Influencing Health Status and Contact with Health Services

OBJECTIVES

After completing this lesson, you should be able to do the following:

- Understand the appropriate uses of codes in this chapter of the ICD-10-CM code book
- Apply knowledge of current, approved ICD-10-CM coding guidelines to assign and sequence accurate codes for diagnoses requiring Z codes
- Identify the main terms in the Alphabetic Index, where common problems or circumstances of admission or encounters are indexed

ICD-10-CM Z Codes

The following blocks represent the ICD-10-CM codes of Chapter 21:

Z00–Z13	Persons encountering health services for examinations
Z14–Z15	Genetic carrier and genetic susceptibility to disease
Z16	Resistance to antimicrobial drugs
Z17	Estrogen receptor status
Z18	Retained foreign body fragment
Z20–Z28	Persons with potential health hazards related to communicable diseases
Z30–Z39	Persons encountering health services in circumstances related to reproduction
Z40–Z53	Encounters for other specific health care
Z55–Z65	Persons with potential health hazards related to socioeconomic and psychosocial circumstances
Z66	Do not resuscitate status

Z67	Blood type
Z68	Body mass index (BMI)
Z69–Z76	Persons encountering health services in other circumstances
Z77–Z99	Persons with potential health hazards related to family and personal history and certain conditions influencing health status

Categories Z00–Z99 are included in the ICD-10-CM code book in Chapter 21, entitled Factors influencing health status and contact with health services. This chapter is useful for coding in the following situations:

- When a person who is currently well uses health services for a specific purpose, such as acting as a donor or receiving prophylactic vaccination

    EXAMPLE: Physician office visit for prophylactic flu shot:

    Z23 Encounter for immunization

- When a circumstance or problem influences the patient's current illness or injury but is not in itself a current illness or injury

    EXAMPLE: Patient visits physician's office complaining of chest pain due to an undetermined cause. The patient is status post open-heart surgery for mitral valve replacement, six months ago:

    R07.9 Chest pain, unspecified

    Z95.2 Presence of prosthetic heart valve

As shown in the preceding example, this Z code is assigned as an additional code.

- When a person with a known disease or injury uses the healthcare system for specific treatment of that disease or injury

    EXAMPLE: Patient visits the clinic for chemotherapy for diagnosis of acute lymphocytic leukemia:

    Z51.11 Encounter for antineoplastic chemotherapy

    C91.00 Acute lymphoblastic leukemia

- To indicate the outcome of delivery

    EXAMPLE: Z37.0 Single live birth

- When a patient has a history, health status, or some other type of problem that is not an injury or illness but it somehow influences the patient's care

    EXAMPLE: Family history

    Personal history of neoplasm

    Personal history of specified diseases

Z codes are sometimes are used in the inpatient hospital setting but more frequently are assigned in the outpatient setting, such as physicians' offices, clinics, or outpatient hospital departments. Moreover, third-party payers may reject some Z codes in claims submitted for payment. A thorough understanding of which Z codes are acceptable or payable will aid in prompt and appropriate payment.

Main Terms

Z codes are indexed in the Alphabetic Index, along with all the other diseases, conditions, symptoms, and so on. However, coders must familiarize themselves with the main terms, where common problems or circumstances are indexed. They should look for terms that describe the reason for the encounter or admission.

> **EXAMPLE:** Patient is seen for closure of a colostomy:
>
> Z43.3 Attention to colostomy

The statement in the preceding example requires a Z code, because the patient was admitted for attention to an artificial opening.

The following main terms included in the Alphabetic Index lead to V codes:

Admission (encounter)	**History (personal) of**
Aftercare	**Maintenance**
Attention to	**Maladjustment**
Boarder	**Newborn**
Care (of)	**Observation**
Carrier (suspected) of	**Outcome of delivery**
Checking	**Problem**
Contact	**Prophylactic**
Contraception, contraceptive	**Replacement by artificial or mechanical device**
Counseling	**or prosthesis of**
Dependence	**Resistance, resistant**
Dialysis	**Screening**
Donor	**Status**
Examination	**Supervision (of)**
Exposure	**Test, Test(s), Testing (for)**
Fitting (of)	**Therapy**
Healthy	**Transplant(ed) Unavailability of medical facilities**
	Vaccination

The main terms listed in the Alphabetic Index are highlighted in boldface type.

Persons Encountering Health Services for Examinations

Categories Z00–Z13 include codes for general, screening, and follow-up examinations. These codes are appropriate for routine visits, especially for preventive care when no complaints are present. In most cases, when a specific condition, sign, or diagnosis is presented and being evaluated, that code should be reported rather than a Z code. Categories Z00–Z13 include the following:

- Z00   Encounter for general examination without complaint, suspected or reported diagnosis
- Z01   Encounter for other special examination without complaints, suspected or reported diagnosis
- Z02   Encounter for administrative examination
- Z03   Encounter for medical observation for suspected diseases and conditions ruled out
- Z04   Encounter for examination and observation for other reason
- Z08   Encounter for follow-up examination after completed treatment for malignant neoplasm
- Z09   Encounter for follow-up examination after completed treatment for conditions other than malignant neoplasm
- Z11   Encounter for screening for infectious and parasitic diseases
- Z12   Encounter for screening for malignant neoplasm
- Z13   Encounter for screening for other diseases and disorders

Categories Z00–Z13 have an Excludes1 note, which excludes examinations related to pregnancy and reproduction.

Genetic Carrier and Genetic Susceptibility to Disease

Codes in category Z14, Genetic carrier, are intended to describe a patient who is known to carry a particular gene that could cause a disease to be passed on to his or her children. The code does not mean that the patient has this particular disease. It does not mean there is 100 percent certainty that the disease would be passed on genetically to the next generation. The code could be used to explain why a patient is receiving additional monitoring or testing.

Codes in category Z15, Genetic susceptibility to disease, are intended to describe a patient who has a confirmed abnormal gene that makes that patient more susceptible to a particular disease. A patient who has a genetic susceptibility to a disease, particularly if it is a malignancy, may request prophylactic removal of an organ to prevent the disease from occurring. For example, code Z40.01, Prophylactic organ removal—breast, would be used in such an encounter followed by the code Z15.01, Genetic susceptibility to malignant neoplasm of breast. Codes from Z15 should not be used as a first-listed code.

Resistance to Antimicrobial Drugs

Category Z16, Resistance to antimicrobial drugs, is provided for us as an additional code(s) to identify the resistance and nonresistance of a specified condition to antimicrobial drugs. There is a note following category Z16 that alerts the coder to "code first the infection."

The subcategory codes identified at the fourth character level are as follows:

- Z16.1 Resistance to beta lactam antibiotics
- Z16.2 Resistance to other antibiotics
- Z16.3 Resistance to other antimicrobial drugs

Estrogen Receptor Status

The status code Z17.0, Estrogen receptor positive status (ER+), or Z17.1, Estrogen receptor negative status (ER−), is used as an additional code for patients who have been diagnosed with breast cancer, both females and males, and have had their estrogen receptor status determined.

About two-thirds of breast cancer patients have an ER+ tumor. The incidence is greater among postmenopausal women. These patients are more likely to benefit from endocrine therapy, so knowledge of their receptor status is important in the selection of adjuvant or palliative therapy. Oral hormones, such as tamoxifen, and estrogen ablation by oophorectomy have proven effective to prolong the duration of disease-free survival, as well as for palliation in the patient with advanced disease when the patient's tumor was ER+.

Retained Foreign Body Fragments

Category Z18, Retained foreign body fragments, outlines several codes that identify specific types of foreign bodies that are retained, such as retained radioactive fragments (Z18.0-), retained metal fragments (Z18.1-), retained plastic fragments (Z18.2), retained organic fragments (Z18.3-), and other and unspecified retained foreign body fragments (Z18.8- and Z18.9).

Persons with Potential Health Hazards Related to Communicable Diseases

Categories Z20–Z28, Persons with potential health hazards related to communicable diseases, include codes that describe patients who have come in contact with, or been exposed to, a communicable disease and who are in need of prophylactic vaccination and inoculation against a disease. The codes in these categories are referenced in the Alphabetic Index under Contact, Exposure, Carrier, Suspected Carrier, Colonization, Prophylactic, and Vaccination.

EXAMPLE: Exposure to rubella:

Z20.4 Contact with and (suspected) exposure to rubella

EXAMPLE: Vaccination against diphtheria:

Z23 Encounter for immunization

Reporting *exposure to* codes may justify the need for services provided to both symptomatic and asymptomatic patients with negative test results.

EXAMPLE: Colonization with MRSA

Z22.322 Carrier or suspected carrier of Methicillin resistant *Staphylococcal aureus* (MRSA colonization)

Codes within these categoies recognize carrier status for typhoid, diphtheria, specific bacterial diseases, viral hepatitis, and diseases with a predominant sexual mode transmission. Some of the commonly used codes in this category are Z22.330, Group B *Streptococcus* carrier; Z22.321, Methicillin susceptible *Staphylococcus aureus* (MSSA) carrier; Z22.322, Methicillin resistant *Staphylococcus aureus* (MRSA) carrier; and Z22.52, Hepatitis C carrier. Many hospitals test patients routinely for MRSA colonization by performing a nasal swab test upon admission that can identify positive or negative MRSA colonization in the patient.

The status codes in category Z22 indicate that the patient is either a carrier or suspected carrier of an infectious disease but currently does not exhibit the symptoms of the disease.

Persons Encountering Health Services in Circumstances Related to Reproduction

Categories Z30–Z39, Persons encountering health services in circumstances related to reproduction, include codes that describe the pregnant state, newborns, supervision of normal and high-risk pregnancy, supervision or care of an infant, postpartum care, contraceptive management, sterilization, procreative management, outcome of delivery, genetic counseling, and antenatal screening.

This section can be further divided into the following categories:

Encounter for Contraceptive Management

Category Z30 includes codes that describe contraceptive management, such as general contraceptive counseling and advice, insertion of intrauterine contraceptive device, encounter for contraceptive counseling and prescription, and surveillance of previously prescribed contraceptive methods. Codes from this category are indexed in the Alphabetic Index under contraception, contraceptive; and sterilization, admission for. Code Z30.2, Sterilization, is assigned as an additional diagnosis when a sterilization procedure is performed during the same admission as a delivery. It may also be assigned as a principal diagnosis when the admission is solely for sterilization. Code Z30.02, Counseling and instruction in natural family planning to avoid pregnancy, is used for those encounters related to natural methods of birth regulation.

Encounter for Procreative Management

Category Z31, Encounter for procreative management, describes healthcare services related to producing an offspring. Services related to reversal of previous sterilization, fertility testing, genetic testing for disease carrier status, genetic counseling, advice using natural family planning, and encounters for Rh incompatibility status and fertility preservation procedures. For example, a couple may be tested either preconception or early in pregnancy to determine carrier status. If both partners are carriers, different pregnancy management may be instituted. Such testing can be performed for cystic fibrosis, Canvan disease, hemoglobinopathies, and Tay-Sachs disease. Because most of the individuals are noncarriers, it is inappropriate to use disease codes to describe the testing encounter; instead, code Z31.430 is used to identify the testing of the female partner, or code Z31.440 is used to identify the testing of the male partner for genetic disease carrier status.

Code Z31.62, reflects encounters for fertility preservation counseling prior to cancer therapy or surgical removal of gonads. Code Z31.83 is used for patients undergoing in vitro fertilization. Code Z31.84 refers to the actual encounter for fertility preservation procedures.

Encounter for Pregnancy Test, Childbirth, and Childcare Instruction

Category Z32 is for encounters for pregnancy tests (positive and negative results) and for childbirth and childcare instructions and includes encounters for prenatal or postpartum care instruction.

Pregnant State

Category Z33 is used to indicate an incidental or not otherwise specified pregnant state. Code Z33.2 is used for those encounters for the elective termination of pregnancy. Code Z33.1 refers to the incidental pregnant state.

Encounter for Supervision of Normal Pregnancy

Category Z34 includes codes for supervision of a normal pregnancy. Generally, codes Z34.0-, Supervision of normal first pregnancy, and Z34.8-, Supervision of other normal pregnancy, are used in the outpatient setting. These codes are referenced in the Alphabetic Index under pregnancy, supervision (of) (for). Fourth character level codes identify the first, second, third, or unspecified trimester of pregnancy.

Encounter for Antenatal Screening of Mother

Category Z36, Encounter for antenatal screening of mother, contains codes for the weeks of gestation (Z3A). These codes are to be used only on the maternal record, and they indicate the weeks of gestation of the pregnancy and are divided as follows:

- Z3A.0 Weeks of gestation of pregnancy, unspecified or less than 10 weeks
- Z3A.1 Weeks of gestation of pregnancy, weeks 10–19
- Z3A.2 Weeks of gestation of pregnancy, weeks 20–29
- Z3A.3 Weeks of gestation of pregnancy, weeks 30–39
- Z3A.4 Weeks of gestation of pregnancy, weeks 40 or greater

Fifth character codes specify the exact week of gestation of the pregnancy.

Outcome of Delivery

Category Z37, Outcome of delivery, contains codes that should be assigned on the mother's health record to indicate whether the outcome of delivery was single or multiple and liveborn or stillborn. The codes in this category are referenced in the Alphabetic Index under Outcome of delivery.

Liveborn Infants According to Place of Birth and Type of Delivery

A code from category Z38, Liveborn infants according to place of birth and type of delivery, is used to identify each type of birth and is always the first code listed on a newborn's health record. The categories describe single or multiple live births, and single or multiple stillbirths. Codes for these categories are located in the Alphabetic Index under Newborn. Any disease or birth injury also should be coded as additional diagnoses, when applicable.

Fourth character codes indicate the following:

.0—Single liveborn infant, born in hospital
.1—Single liveborn infant, born outside hospital
.2—Single liveborn infant, unspecified as to place of birth
.3—Twin liveborn infant, born in hospital
.4—Twin liveborn infant, born outside hospital
.5—Twin liveborn infant, unspecified as to place of birth
.6—Other multiple liveborn infant, born in hospital
.7—Other multiple liveborn infant, born outside hospital
.8—Other multiple liveborn infant, unspecified as to place of birth

Fifth character codes indicate the following:

0—Delivered vaginally
1—Delivered by cesarean

Encounter for Maternal Postpartum Care and Examination

Category Z39, Encounter for maternal postpartum care and examination, is used in the following situations:

- For the care and examination of mother immediately after delivery, when such delivery occurs outside the healthcare facility;
- For care and examination of lactating mother and for supervision of lactating mother
- For routine postpartum follow-up

Encounters for Other Specific Health Care

The following note appears at the beginning of categories Z40–Z53, Encounter for other specific health care: "categories Z40–Z53 are intended for use to indicate a reason for care in patients who may have already been treated for some disease or injury not now present, or who are receiving care or prophylactic care, or care to consolidate the treatment, to deal with a residual state." The section is subdivided to describe the type of service provided. Codes in categories Z40–Z53 are indexed in the Alphabetic Index under admission (encounter), for aftercare; attention to; dialysis; and donor.

For encounters specifically for prophylactic removal of breasts, ovaries, or another organ due to risk factors related to malignant neoplasms, the principal or first-listed code should be a code from category Z40, Encounter for prophylactic surgery, followed by the appropriate risk factor code.

Other conditions indexed under this section include the following:

- Plastic and reconstructive surgery following a medical procedure or healed injury
- Attention to artificial openings
- Fitting and adjustment of external prosthetic devices and other devices
- Adjustment and management of implanted device
- Orthopedic aftercare and other postprocedural aftercare
- Care involving renal dialysis
- Other aftercare
- Donors of organs and tissues
- Specific procedures and treatment not carried out

Persons with Potential Health Hazards Related to Socioeconomic and Psychosocial Circumstances

Persons with potential hazards related to socioeconomic and psychosocial circumstances include the following specific categories:

- Z55 Problems related to education and literacy
- Z56 Problems related to employment and unemployment
- Z57 Occupational exposure to risk factors
- Z59 Problems related to housing and economic circumstances
- Z60 Problems related to social environment
- Z62 Problems related to upbringing
- Z63 Other problems related to primary support group, including family circumstances
- Z64 Problems related to certain psychosocial circumstances
- Z65 Problems related to other psychosocial circumstances

This section contains circumstances that in some cases will impact a patient's medical or emotional condition. Some examples include divorce or legal separations, parent-child estrangements, and loss of job.

Do Not Resuscitate

ICD-10-CM has a separate category exclusively for *do not resuscitate* or DNR status. Today, more and more patients are indicating their wishes with this type of status listed on their health record.

Blood Type

Category Z67 in ICD-10-CM delineates a person's blood type (A, B, AB, O), which is identified at the fourth character level. Fifth characters designate whether the type is positive or negative.

Body Mass Index

The body mass index (BMI) is the first determination of a patient's weight in proportion to height. BMI measures are calculated as kilograms per meters squared. The adult BMI codes are for use with individuals older than 20 years. Codes in this category were created to be used in conjunction with a code from E66, Overweight and obesity, to provide specific information about a patient's weight. BMI codes are also used when a code is reported for a diagnosis of underweight (R63.6) or loss of weight (R63.4). Codes that specify specific ranges for the adult BMI are Z68.2- through Z68.4-. Pediatric BMI codes (Z68.5-) are for use for persons age 2 to 20 years.

For the BMI, code assignment may be based on medical record documentation from clinicians who are not the patient's provider (that is, physician or other qualified healthcare practitioner legally accountable for establishing the patient's diagnosis), since this information is typically documented by other clinicians involved in the care of the patient (for example, a dietitian or nurse). However, the associated diagnosis (such as overweight or obesity) must be documented by the patient's provider.

Persons Encountering Health Services in Other Circumstances

In ICD-10-CM, categories Z69-Z76, Persons encountering health services in other circumstances, include codes for the following type of conditions or situations:

- Z69   Mental health services for victim and perpetrator of abuse (includes parental child abuse, non-parental child abuse and spouse or partner abuse)
- Z70   Counseling related to sexual attitude, behavior and orientation (includes patient's sexual behavior and orientation, and sex counseling)
- Z71   Other counseling and medical advice, not elsewhere classified (includes dietarycounseling, alcohol and drug abuse counseling and tobacco counseling)
- Z72   Problems related to lifestyle (includes tobacco use, high risk sexual behavior, lack of physical exercise, inappropriate diet, and eating habits, gambling and betting, sleep deprivation)
- Z73   Problems related to life management difficulty (includes burnout stress, NEC, inadequate social skills, childhood behavioral insomnia)
- Z74   Problems related to care provider dependency (includes reduced mobility, need for assistance with personal care and continuous supervision)
- Z75   Problems related to medical facilities and other health care (includes holiday relief care, awaiting admission to adequate facilities elsewhere, medical services not available in home)
- Z76   Persons encountering health services in other circumstances (includes issue of repeat prescription, healthy person accompanying sick person, awaiting organ transplant status, health supervision and care of foundling)

Persons with Potential Health Hazards Related to Family and Personal History and Certain Conditions Influencing Health Status

Categories Z77 – Z99, Persons with potential health hazards related to family and personal history and certain conditions influencing health status, have a note immediately following the category to "code also any follow-up examination."

Codes in categories Z77–Z79 include the following:

- Contact with and (suspected) exposures hazardous to health
- Exposure to environmental pollution
- Asymptomatic menopausal state
- Physical restraint status
- Long-term (current) drug therapy (includes anticoagulants, hormonal contraception, insulin, steroids, drug therapy, hormone replacement therapy)

Another part of this section (categories Z80–Z87) contains codes related to family and personal history. The family history codes may be important to note, as some diseases or conditions are hereditary, and it would be extremely useful for the physician to be aware of this for patient monitoring purposes. Codes are included for conditions such as neoplasms, mental and behavioral disorders, heart disease, arthritis, HIV, endocrine and metabolic disorders, and respiratory conditions.

The personal history codes are equally important, because they identify any malignant neoplasms the patient may have had. Personal history codes are provided for various body systems, and certain other diseases such as *in situ* and benign neoplasms, infectious and parasitic diseases, and various other disease processes that present in the various systems of the body.

Category Z89 refers to the acquired absence of limbs and organs not elsewhere classified. Category Z91 refers to personal risk factors, such as allergy to things other than drugs and biological substances, such as peanuts, milk products, eggs, and seafood. Also included are personal history codes including adult abuse, self-harm, contraception, and irradiation. Category Z93 identifies artificial opening status such as tracheostomy and colostomy, while category Z94 codes are status codes for transplanted organs and tissues.

The presence of cardiac and vascular implants and grafts, as well as other functional implants, are coded to categories Z95 and Z96.

Category Z98, Other postprocedural states, includes codes for conditions such as sterilization status, angioplasty status, breast implant status, and dental procedure status. Category Z99 refers to the dependence on enabling machines and devices such as aspirators, respirators, renal dialysis, supplemental oxygen, and wheelchairs.

Codes in all of these sections may or may not be first-listed codes, but in most cases they serve as secondary codes to further explain or identify listed conditions. Those codes may be especially useful for physician office documentation.

Chapter 21: ICD-10-CM Exercises

Review the following statements and assign the appropriate codes:

1. Status post unilateral kidney transplant, human donor

2. Encounter for chemotherapy for patient with Hodgkin's lymphoma

3. Reprogramming of cardiac pacemaker

4. Gastrostomy tube irrigation

5. Encounter for breast augmentation

6. Office visit for gynecological examination, including Pap smear

7. Follow-up examination of colon adenocarcinoma resected one year ago, no recurrence found

8. Encounter for changing a surgical wound dressing

9. Routine general medical examination for an adult

10. Encounter for paternity testing

11. Tetanus vaccination

12. Patient presenting for a routine screening mammogram due to a strong family history of breast cancer

13. Encounter for sterilization

14. Encounter for fertility testing

15. Screening for developmental handicap for a two-year-old child

16. Encounter for ear piercing

17. Gastric bypass status for obesity

18. This single newborn was born vaginally in the hospital. The baby is being treated for Rh incompatibility in a baby with documented type A+ blood, and the mother's blood type documented as A-. What is the correct diagnosis code(s)?

19. A set of twins were born in the hospital and were delivered by cesarean section. Both of the babies were liveborn. How would this be coded?

20. Patient seen for fitting of right artificial leg after patient had below-knee amputation due to medical condition.

21. Postmenopausal osteoporosis in a 63-year-old female with a history of healed osteoporotic fracture of the ankle.

22. The patient presents to his physician's office for a medical examination and chest x-ray because he Is scheduled for surgery for chronic cholecystitis. The physician Informs him that his chest x-ray was normal. What are the correct diagnosis codes?

23. The patient is seen by her obstetrician for a pregnancy test. The result of the pregnancy test was negative. How would this be coded?

24. A baby boy was born in the hospital and was immediately diagnosed with a cleft hard palate and a unilateral cleft lip.

Challenges of Compliance and Ethical Coding

After completing this lesson, you should be able to do the following:

- Describe the various federal laws and programs that form the basis for healthcare fraud and abuse initiatives
- Differentiate between fraud and abuse and give examples of each
- Outline the steps in the development of a physician compliance plan

ICD-10-CM

As the largest third-party payer, the Medicare program is the frequent target of fraud and abuse, which costs the government billions of healthcare dollars. Over the past several years, the government has enacted legislation and committed resources (money and people) to fight bilking of the Medicare and Medicaid programs.

Legislation Addressing Fraud and Abuse

A number of federal laws and programs form the basis for prosecution of healthcare fraud and abuse perpetrators. Some of these are as follows:

- The Federal False Claims Act, enacted in 1863, allows a private citizen to sue an individual or a company it believes to be submitting false bills to the federal government. The original intent of this act was to discourage war profiteers who were committing fraud against the Army in the post–Civil War era. In 1986, the Federal False Claims Amendment Act was signed into law by President Reagan. This amendment strengthened the government's ability to prosecute healthcare providers or suppliers who defraud the government. In the original law, there had to be a specific intent to defraud. The amendment removes the intent criterion. It also delineates penalties for each offense that a provider is found guilty of and allows triple damages to be imposed. The act offers financial incentives to informants, or relators, who report providers to the government. This is known as a qui tam action. Furthermore, the law protects the relators from being threatened or harassed in any way by the employer. Relators are awarded between 15 and 30 percent of the total monies recovered.

- The Health Insurance Portability and Accountability Act (HIPAA), enacted in 1996 by President Clinton, has several significant provisions establishing expanded fraud and abuse controls. HIPAA strengthened the jurisdiction of the Department of Health and Human Services (HHS) and increased the investigative powers and funding available to the Office of the Inspector General (OIG) and the FBI for healthcare fraud and abuse controls. HIPAA provides for criminal penalties for healthcare professionals who knowingly and willfully attempt to defraud any of the healthcare benefit programs. It also provides for imprisonment for violators. Furthermore, this legislation stipulates that physicians or other providers are accountable for information they know or should know. This means that if an issue was addressed in an official source, such as *ICD-10-CM Official Guidelines for Coding and Reporting*, it is expected that the physician should have known it. When ICD-10-CM becomes law, the same is true for those coding guidelines.

- In 2009, President Obama signed into law the Fraud Enforcement and Recovery Act, which made it easier for CMS and law enforcement agencies to go after those committing healthcare fraud. The Health Care Fraud Prevention and Enforcement Action Team was revamped as an interagency program that works to improve existing fraud detection programs, using technology to stop fraudulent activity before payment is rendered. The Health Information Technology for Economic and Clinical Health Act (HITECH) was passed in 2009 and also strengthened the penalties awarded to healthcare facilities found in violation of fraud and abuse laws.

- Operation Restore Trust, enacted in 1995, is a HHS program that involves federal and state government officials and private-sector representatives. The project is designed to combat fraud and abuse through various initiatives. Several million dollars of overpayments have been recouped, and numerous criminal convictions and civil judgments have been handed down as a result of Operation Restore Trust.

- The Balanced Budget Act of 1997 includes 15 sections on fraud and abuse and gives government agencies additional tools in the fight to control healthcare costs.

- One of the new fraud and abuse detection initiatives is the Zone Program Integrity Contractor (ZPIC) program. ZPIC was developed out of the Program Safeguard Contractors (PSCs) program, which was created in 1999 to detect fraud in the various CMS benefit plans. While the PSCs searched for fraud in only one benefit plan each, such as Part A, Part B, or Home Health, the ZPICs will search all CMS benefit plans for signs of fraudulent behavior.

- Stark Legislation (Stark I, II, and III) is a limitation on certain referrals of designated health service to facilities in which the provider has a financial interest. The original Stark law addressed concerns with laboratory services, but subsequent laws (Stark II and III) expanded this to other healthcare organizations such as imaging centers, physical therapy offices, or durable medical equipment (DME) companies.

In addition to these federal laws and programs, many states have legislation and programs designed to combat fraud and abuse. States are particularly active in the prosecution of Medicaid false claims.

Agencies Involved in Investigating Fraud and Abuse

Several government agencies actually participate in the war against fraud and abuse. The OIG investigates and prosecutes individuals who over-bill Medicare. It also develops an annual work plan that delineates the specific target areas that will be monitored in a given year.

The FBI is the principal investigative arm of the Department of Justice and conducts civil and criminal fraud investigations. The Postal Inspection Service has authority to investigate fraudulent schemes involving the US Postal Service. The Defense Criminal Investigative Service (DCIS) is responsible for investigating potential fraud against the government's military healthcare plans. The US Attorneys' offices and state attorney generals also are involved in prosecuting violators.

Definitions and Examples of Fraud and Abuse

Medicare defines fraud as an intentional deception or misrepresentation that results in an unauthorized benefit to an individual. Fraud may take many forms, including the following:

- Billing for services or supplies that were not provided, which may include phantom billing or ghost billing for patients who were not seen by the provider
- Altering claim forms or medical records to obtain higher reimbursement than is appropriate
- Receiving kickbacks in exchange for referring patients to specific facilities
- Misrepresenting the types of services provided, dates of services, or even the identity of the patient
- Billing for noncovered services
- Billing for gang visits, which is billing for visits to multiple patients (for example, in a nursing home) when no specific services were provided
- Billing for equipment that was never provided

Abuse involves billing practices that are inconsistent with generally acceptable fiscal policies. This usually results from inadvertent coding or billing mistakes and is not considered fraudulent.

Physician Compliance

One way that physicians can prevent or minimize potentially abusive or fraudulent activities is through the development of a compliance plan. The OIG has published a model compliance plan for small and individual physician practices. This document delineates seven basic steps, or program guidelines.

Model Compliance Plan
Step 1. Institute Auditing and Monitoring
The OIG contends that an audit is an invaluable tool for a physician practice to determine what, if any, problem areas exist. Any problems that are encountered can be addressed with corrective measures. Periodic auditing of billing practices to determine that the documentation in the record supports the services billed, that medical necessity guidelines are followed, and that bills are coded correctly is an essential part of the compliance puzzle. An initial baseline audit should be undertaken to give the practice a benchmark against which to measure future results.

Step 2. Implement Written Policies, Procedures, and Standards of Conduct
In developing policies and procedures, the physician should be aware of the risk areas that the OIG has identified for physician practices. These include the following:

- Coding and billing: AHIMA has established the AHIMA Code of Ethics and Standards of Ethical Coding that can be used as the basis for a healthcare facility's code of conduct
- Certification of need for DME and home health services

- Documentation in the medical record
- Billing for noncovered services as if they are covered
- Up-coding (billing for a more expensive service than the one actually performed)
- Unbundling
- Clustering (coding or charging one or two middle levels of service codes exclusively)

Step 3. Designate a Compliance Officer or Contact to Monitor Compliance Efforts

The individual designated to monitor compliance efforts may be the office manager, the practice administrator, the billing supervisor, or an outside consultant or consulting firm. Responsibilities of the position might include the following:

- Overseeing and monitoring implementation of the compliance program
- Establishing methods, such as audits, to improve the practice's efficiency and quality of services and to reduce its vulnerability to fraud and abuse charges
- Periodically revising the compliance program in light of changes in government and third-party rules and regulations
- Developing, coordinating, and participating in training programs
- Ensuring that the HHS, OIG's List of Excluded Individuals and Entities, and the General Services Administration's List of Parties Debarred from Federal Programs have been checked with respect to all employees, medical staff, and independent contractors
- Investigating reports or allegations concerning possible unethical or improper business practices

Step 4. Develop Training and Educational Programs

Training and educational programs may take several forms, including in-house training sessions or outside seminars and workshops, and may be supplemented by written newsletters with coding tips or bulletin boards. Up to date coding books, newsletters, and reference materials should be made available for office personnel. Moreover, the physician practice should offer both initial and recurrent training in compliance. The training might address the operation and importance of the compliance program, consequences of violating the practice's standards and procedures, and the employees' role in the program's operation. Training in specific coding guidelines and billing practices also is necessary.

Step 5. Respond Appropriately to Detected Violations

When offenses are discovered, they should be investigated and corrective measures undertaken. Physician practices should develop indicators that would signal a problem. These might include the following:

- A significant change in the number of claim rejections or reduction in payments
- Changes in the pattern of Current Procedural Terminology code usage
- Increased number of challenges to the medical necessity of services provided

Corrective actions may include refunding overpayments from a third-party payer or even self-reporting to the government.

Step 6. Develop Open Lines of Communication to Keep Practice Employees Updated about Compliance Activities

Open lines of communication may be accomplished through suggestion boxes, bulletin boards, hot lines, an established open door policy between the physician or compliance officer and the employees, and discussions at staff meetings.

Step 7. Enforce Disciplinary Standards through Thoroughly Published Guidelines

Disciplinary action may take several forms, including oral warnings, written reprimands, probation or demotion, suspension, termination, or referral for criminal prosecution.

A well-established compliance program can assist a physician practice in developing and implementing controls and procedures that will ensure adherence to federal healthcare programs and other third-party payer requirements.

Summary

The challenges facing the coding and billing personnel in the physician office setting are numerous. A thorough knowledge of ICD-10-CM coding guidelines as well as access to various coding resources, such as *ICD-10-CM Official Guidelines for Coding and Reporting* and authoritative resources from the American Hospital Association (such as *Coding Clinic*), are essential to accurate coding and billing. Physicians should be aware of the government and private sector initiatives to combat fraud and abuse and diligently monitor their reimbursement practices to meet the requirements of third-party payers. Establishment of a compliance program, including requirements for continuing education of the reimbursement personnel, will assist the physician practice in adhering to private-sector and government rules and regulations.

Training and Implementation of ICD-10-CM

Lessons Learned from Other Nations

Both Australia and Canada have developed modifications of ICD-10 for use in their countries. ICD-10-AM and ICD-10-CA were developed with the permission of the World Health Organization (WHO), as was ICD-10-CM. ICD-10-AM has been fully implemented in Australia since 1999, and most of Canada has completed the conversion to ICD-10-CA. In both countries, implementation was phased in over the course of two years. Canada has an entirely electronic ICD-10-CA product; no printed ICD-10-CA code books are available. Australia and Canada adopted ICD-10 because of the need for a more clinically useful case-mix index and also because of its applicability in nonacute care settings.

In Australia, the National Center for Classification in Health (NCCH) formed an ICD-10-AM Education Working Party composed of individuals from educational facilities, professional organizations, and NCCH Education Division staff. Between 1995 and 1999, the NCCH conducted training courses and developed educational materials. In addition, postimplementation workshops were held to clarify coding issues.

The NCCH prepared and distributed ICD-10-AM implementation kits to all healthcare facilities. These kits included information briefing (fact) sheets and visual aids on topics such as the background behind the move to ICD-10-AM, details about the classification system, stages of the implementation process, and information on transitional issues. In addition, the NCCH released six booklets on various topics related to implementing the new system.

Canada provided coding education in a three-phase plan. The first phase was a self-learning package that required about 21 hours to complete. The second phase consisted of a two-day workshop, with a hands-on program. In the third phase, a self-learning package of 10 case studies was provided to users. All of the education in Canada involved the use of coding software and not code books. Both countries offer periodic refresher courses. The average learning curve was four to six months, and users reported that they did not find ICD-10 any more or less difficult to learn than ICD-9 (Prophet 2002).

Training in the United States

Obviously, coding professionals and physicians will require training, but other individuals will also be affected and need some training, depending on the extent of their involvement.

Educational efforts may take many forms. Face-to-face workshops or seminars will continue to be an important part of any type of retraining program, but there are several alternatives for individuals who cannot travel to a seminar or workshop. Currently, a number of excellent coding publications are dedicated to coding training. The American Health Information Management Association (AHIMA) and other organizations have tools for coding training available now and more will be added each year as the implementation date, October 1, 2014, approaches. AHIMA's Train the Trainer programs have educated several thousand HIM professionals. Audio seminars that deliver information to a large audience are cost effective, because no travel is involved. Certainly, web-based training will play an important role. Many vendors already have excellent coding programs available that presumably will be adapted to ICD-10-CM. Web-based training is particularly useful in training large numbers of individuals and can be highly effective, depending on the quality of the program and the dedication of the participants.

Educators in coding certificate programs, health information technology programs, and health information administration programs will be charged with the task of training new coding professionals. Professional associations such as AHIMA will take the lead in retraining the coding professionals in the workforce through continuing education programs.

Training for Coding Professionals

Although ICD-10-CM is different from ICD-9-CM in many ways, the new classification system retains the traditional format and many of the same characteristics and conventions. Thus, experienced coding professionals should have little difficulty in achieving coding proficiency. Experienced coding professionals will require education on changes in the structure of the codes, definitions, and guidelines. There are many more trained coding professionals today as compared to when ICD-9-CM was introduced, but less experienced users will face a number of challenges. The increased level of specificity with ICD-10-CM will require a strong foundation in anatomy and physiology, medical terminology, pharmacology, and medical science. Assessing the need for additional training in these areas is important. AHIMA's recommendation for training on coding is:

- 50 hours total
  - ▶ 16 for ICD-10-CM
  - ▶ 24 for PCS
  - ▶ 10 hands-on practice

Training for Physicians

The inadequacy of physician documentation has been an obstacle to complete and accurate coding for years. With the increased specificity in ICD-10-CM, complete documentation will be a factor in the collection of accurate statistical data as well as the key to appropriate reimbursement. A careful review of the code changes for ICD-10-CM clearly demonstrates the necessity of complete documentation and the use of current terminology. Having physicians actively involved in the implementation process allows them the opportunity to understand the importance of complete and accurate health record documentation.

Documentation assessment will continue to be an important tool for improving physician documentation. Results of the assessments can be shared with the physicians, and instances where patient care was compromised or revenue was lost because of inadequate documentation can be highlighted. Information on the uses of coded data apart from reimbursement should be shared with physicians as well, so that they can better understand the impact of documentation.

Training for Other Healthcare Professionals

Many users of health record data will require varying levels of training, depending on their involvement with coded data. Some of these users include the following:

- Clinicians other than physicians, such as nurses and allied health professionals
- Quality management personnel
- Utilization management and case management personnel
- Data quality and data security personnel
- Researchers, data analysts, and epidemiologists
- Software vendors
- Information systems personnel
- Billing, decision support, and accounting personnel
- Compliance officers
- Internal and external auditors and consulting firms
- Fraud investigators
- Government agency personnel, including recovery audit contractors

Impact on Information Systems

The move to ICD-10-CM might be compared to the anticipated collapse of computer systems worldwide at the change of the century (known as Y2K) in the amount of work faced by information systems personnel. All electronic transactions requiring a diagnosis or procedure code will need to be reviewed, and possibly changed. Some of the various systems that will need to be reviewed include billing systems, decision support systems, clinical systems, encoding software, health record abstracting systems, aggregate data reporting, utilization and quality management systems, case-mix systems, accounting systems, clinical protocols, test ordering systems, clinical reminder systems, performance measurement systems, medical necessity software, and benefits determination.

Software will need to be developed to accommodate field size expansion, alphanumeric codes, redefinitions of code values, edit and logic changes, modifications of table structure, and expansion of flat files containing diagnosis codes and systems interfaces. Specific examples include the following:

- Any field that requires a code will need to accommodate up to seven characters rather than five.
- Any field that requires a code will need to be changed to accept alphanumeric codes in addition to numeric codes (this may not be an issue because of the V codes and E codes already used in ICD-9-CM).
- ICD-10-CM codes may have up to four characters (numbers or letters) after the decimal point. In ICD-9-CM, there is a maximum of only two numbers after the decimal point.
- The size of data fields accommodating descriptions of the codes may have to be reviewed. Code titles are much more descriptive and, thus, longer in ICD-10-CM than in ICD-9-CM.
- ICD-10-CM offers many more codes than ICD-9-CM does. Therefore, the systems used by healthcare organizations will need to be able to accommodate additional data. Both ICD-9-CM and ICD-10-CM will have to be supported by the computer hardware.
- ICD-10-CM codes that consist of five characters may be confused with Healthcare Common Procedure Coding System Level II codes, which also begin with an alphabetic character. This will not be a problem if the decimal point is placed in the ICD-10-CM codes, but it might be a problem if the software did not use the decimal.

Impact on Budgeting and Reimbursement

In order to gauge the impact of implementing ICD-10-CM and ICD-10-PCS in any specific facility, the organization's chief financial officer will need to look at capital expenditures such as new or upgraded hardware, new software, training costs for coding professionals and other personnel, and finally, the hiring of information systems personnel to accomplish the changeover.

In addition, there will likely be delays in payments from third-party payers until coders and billing personnel are fully trained on the system. A learning curve will exist for the coders when they first start using ICD-10-CM. An expected loss of productivity will have to be considered. Moreover, there may be an increased number of claims denials or rejections due to inadequate coding, reporting, and processing. Initially, payments should not be substantially affected from the standpoint of reimbursement systems. CMS will be providing the general equivalence mappings (GEMs) files, which are a public domain reference mapping designed to provide all sectors of the healthcare industry that use coded data with a tool to convert and test systems, link data in long term clinical studies, develop application-specific mappings, and analyze data collected during the transition period and beyond. However, there are many areas that the GEMs cannot address, given the much greater number of ICD-10-CM codes. At some point, managed care contracts and negotiated rate schedules will be recalculated using ICD-10-CM data.

Eventually, ICD-10-CM data will allow for more robust data analysis because of its specificity and provide the predicted following benefits:

- Allow for appropriate refinements of reimbursement systems to better reflect the actual cost of patient care
- Improve providers' and payers' ability to negotiate reimbursement rates
- Improve payers' ability to forecast healthcare needs and analyze healthcare costs
- Reduce payers' and providers' costs due to improved ability to do the following:

  ‣ Effectively monitor service and resource utilization
  ‣ Analyze healthcare costs
  ‣ Monitor outcomes
  ‣ Measure performance
  ‣ Detect fraud and abuse

Moreover, the increased specificity should reduce the number of requests for health records to justify payment, because the codes should provide the information needed.

Amount and Timing of Training

In 2003, AHIMA and the American Health Association conducted field testing of the ICD-10-CM medical code sets. The study showed ICD-10-CM to be a significant improvement over the current ICD-9-CM coding system, and ICD-10-CM can be implemented without excessive staff training costs or changes in documentation practices. Training ICD-9-CM users to use ICD-10-CM was shown to be relatively straightforward, because ICD-10-CM retains the traditional ICD format and many of the same conventions.

As part of the ICD-10-CM Field Testing Project, participants who coded the same records with ICD-9-CM and with ICD-10-CM were asked how many hours of ICD-10-CM training they thought they would need prior to implementation. The majority (60 percent) indicated they would need 16 hours of training or less. Another 24 percent indicated they would need 17 to 24 hours of training. This estimate is less than what the Department of Health and Human Services (HHS) estimated in the Final Rule published on January 16, 2009, for the HIPAA Administrative Simplification: Modification to the Medical Data Code Set Standards to Adopt ICD-10-CM and

ICD-10-PCS in which the HHS estimated the need of 50 hours for hospital inpatient coders to learn both ICD-9-CM and ICD-10-PCS. For outpatient or physician-based coders, the HHS estimated the need of 10 hours of training to learn ICD-10-CM diagnosis coding. The difference in the estimate between these two settings is learning the procedure coding system, ICD-10-PCS. Because of the significant difference between the ICD-9-CM Volume 3 procedure format and the new ICD-10-PCS organization and structure, it is predicted that the majority of the training time for inpatient coders will be devoted to learning ICD-10-PCS (HHS, 2013).

Again in the ICD-10-CM Field Testing Project, participants were asked when ICD-10-CM and ICD-10-PCS should be provided to coders. The majority of respondents (almost 60 percent) thought that training should be provided three months prior to ICD-10-CM implementation. Another 29 percent of the participants suggested training be conducted six months prior to implementation. Less than 10 percent of the respondents recommended that training be provided for more than one year prior to implementation.

Conclusion

The *International Classification of Diseases, 10th Edition, Clinical Modification* is scheduled to be implemented for the coding of all diagnoses, injuries, and conditions for encounters or discharges occurring on or after October 1, 2014. ICD-10-CM will provide significant improvements through greater detailed information and the ability to expand in order to capture additional advancements in clinical medicine. Furthermore, it will enhance accurate payment for services rendered and facilitate evaluation of medical procedures and outcomes to improve patient care and patient safety.

Readers who are interested in gaining hands-on practice coding in ICD-10-CM and ICD-10-PCS should refer to the AHIMA website and review the many publications related to ICD-10-CM coding.

References and Bibliography

American Diabetes Association. 2013. http://www.diabetes.org.

American Health Information Management Association and the American Hospital Association. 2003. *ICD-10-CM Field Testing Project: Report on findings.* http://www.ahima.org/downloads /pdfs/resources/FinalStudy_000.pdf.

American Hospital Association. 1984–2013. *Coding Clinic for ICD-9-CM.* Chicago, IL: American Hospital Association.

American Psychiatric Association. 2005. *Diagnostic and Statistical Manual of Mental Disorders, Text Revision,* 4th ed. Arlington, VA: American Psychiatric Association.

Berkow, R., M. Burs, and M. Beers, eds. 1999. *Merck Manual of Diagnosis and Therapy,* 18th ed. Rahway, NJ: Merck and Company.

Centers for Medicare and Medicaid Services. 2013. General ICD-10 Information. http://www .cms.hhs.gov/ICD10.

Department of Health and Human Services. 45 CFR Part 162: Administrative Requirements. 2013 (Jan. 25).

Department of Health and Human Services. 2013. *ICD-10-CM Official Guidelines for Coding and Reporting.* http://www.cdc.gov/nchs/data/icd10/10cmguidelines_2013_final.pdf.

DeVault, K., A. Barta, and M. Endicott. 2012. *ICD-10-CM Coder Training Manual,* 2012 ed. Chicago, IL: American Health Information Management Association.

Dorland. 2012. *Dorland's Pocket Medical Dictionary,* 29th ed. Philadelphia, PA: Saunders.

Holt, J.G. 2011. *Bergey's Manual of Systematic Bacteriology,* 2nd ed. Baltimore, MD: Lippincott Williams & Wilkins.

Johnson, S.L. and C.S. McHugh. 2006. *Understanding Medical Coding: A Comprehensive Guide.* Albany, NY: Delmar Publishers.

Leon-Chisen, N. 2013. *ICD-10-CM and ICD-10-PCS Coding Handbook.* Chicago, IL: American Hospital Association.

National Center for Health Statistics. 2013. *International Classification of Diseases, Tenth Revision, Clinical Modification (ICD-10-CM).* http://www.cdc.gov/nchs/icd/icd10cm.htm.

National Pressure Ulcer Advisory Panel. 2007. Pressure Ulcer Category/Staging Illustrations. http://www.npuap.org/resources/.

OptumInsight. 2013. *ICD-10-CM: The Complete Official Draft Code Set.* Salt Lake City, UT: OptumInsight.

Prophet, Sue. 2002. *Testimony of the American Health Information Management Association to the National Committee on Vital and Health Statistics on ICD-10-CM.* http://ncvhs.hhs .gov/020529p05.htm.

Scott, K.S. 2011. *2011 Coding and Reimbursement for Hospital Inpatient Services.* Chicago, IL: American Health Information Management Association.

Schraffenberger, L.A. 2013. *Basic ICD-10-CM/PCS Coding.* Chicago, IL: American Health Information Management Association.

Stedman's. 2006. *Stedman's Medical Dictionary,* 28th ed. Baltimore, MD: Lippincott, Williams, and Wilkins.

Venes, Donald, ed. 2013. *Taber's Cyclopedic Medical Dictionary,* 22nd ed. Philadelphia, PA: F.A. Davis Company.

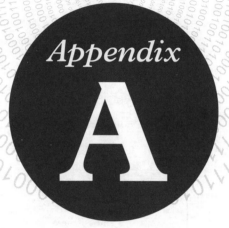

CMS-1500 Claim Form and the ABN Form

The CMS-1500 Health Insurance Claim Form (figure A.1) and 1500 Claim Form Reference Instruction Manual can be accessed at the National Uniform Claim Committee website. On July 2, 2007, Form CMS-1500 (12-90) was discontinued, and only Form CMS-1500 (08-05) is to be used.

The Advance Beneficiary Notice of Noncoverage (ABN) sample form is shown in figure A.2. The revised ABN form may also be used for voluntary notifications in place of the Notice of Exclusions from Medicare Benefits form. The ABN form, form instructions, and Spanish forms are available online at the Centers for Medicare and Medicaid website.

Figure A.1. CMS-1500 Health Insurance Claim Form

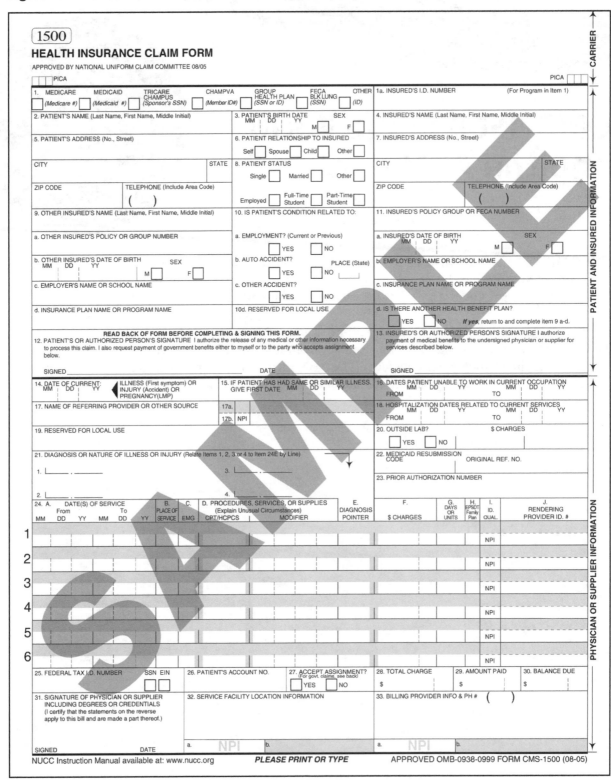

Figure A.2. Advance Beneficiary Notice of Noncoverage

A. Notifier:

B. Patient Name: **C. Identification Number:**

Advance Beneficiary Notice of Noncoverage (ABN)

NOTE: If Medicare doesn't pay for **D.** ———————— below, you may have to pay.
Medicare does not pay for everything, even some care that you or your health care provider have good reason to think you need. We expect Medicare may not pay for the **D.** ———————— below.

D.	E. Reason Medicare May Not Pay:	F. Estimated Cost

WHAT YOU NEED TO DO NOW:
- Read this notice, so you can make an informed decision about your care.
- Ask us any questions that you may have after you finish reading.
- Choose an option below about whether to receive the **D.** ———————— listed above.
  Note: If you choose Option 1 or 2, we may help you to use any other insurance that you might have, but Medicare cannot require us to do this.

G. OPTIONS: Check only one box. We cannot choose a box for you.

☐ **OPTION 1.** I want the **D.** ———————— listed above. You may ask to be paid now, but I also want Medicare billed for an official decision on payment, which is sent to me on a Medicare Summary Notice (MSN). I understand that if Medicare doesn't pay, I am responsible for payment, but **I can appeal to Medicare** by following the directions on the MSN. If Medicare does pay, you will refund any payments I made to you, less co-pays or deductibles.

☐ **OPTION 2.** I want the **D.** ———————— listed above, but do not bill Medicare. You may ask to be paid now as I am responsible for payment. **I cannot appeal if Medicare is not billed**.

☐ **OPTION 3.** I don't want the **D.** ———————— listed above. I understand with this choice I am **not** responsible for payment, and **I cannot appeal to see if Medicare would pay.**

H. Additional Information:

This notice gives our opinion, not an official Medicare decision. If you have other questions on this notice or Medicare billing, call **1-800-MEDICARE** (1-800-633-4227/**TTY:** 1-877-486-2048).
Signing below means that you have received and understand this notice. You also receive a copy.

I. Signature:	J. Date:

According to the Paperwork Reduction Act of 1995, no persons are required to respond to a collection of information unless it displays a valid OMB control number. The valid OMB control number for this information collection is 0938-0566. The time required to complete this information collection is estimated to average 7 minutes per response, including the time to review instructions, search existing data resources, gather the data needed, and complete and review the information collection. If you have comments concerning the accuracy of the time estimate or suggestions for improving this form, please write to: CMS, 7500 Security Boulevard, Attn: PRA Reports Clearance Officer, Baltimore, Maryland 21244-1850.

Form CMS-R-131 (03/11)   Form Approved OMB No. 0938-0566

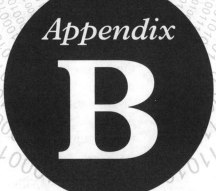

B

AHIMA Standards of Ethical Coding

Introduction

The Standards of Ethical Coding are based on the American Health Information Management Association's (AHIMA's) Code of Ethics. Both sets of principles reflect expectations of professional conduct for coding professionals involved in diagnostic or procedural coding or other health record data abstraction.

A code of ethics sets forth professional values and ethical principles and offers ethical guidelines to which professionals aspire and by which their actions can be judged. Health information management (HIM) professionals are expected to demonstrate professional values by their actions to patients, employers, members of the healthcare team, the public, and the many stakeholders they serve. A code of ethics is important in helping to guide the decision-making process and can be referenced by individuals, agencies, organizations, and other bodies (such as licensing and regulatory boards, insurance providers, courts of law, government agencies, and other professional groups).

The AHIMA Code of Ethics (available on the AHIMA website) is relevant to all AHIMA members and credentialed HIM professionals and students, regardless of their professional functions, the settings in which they work, or the populations they serve. Coding is one of the core HIM functions, and due to the complex regulatory requirements affecting the health information coding process, coding professionals are frequently faced with ethical challenges.

The AHIMA Standards of Ethical Coding are intended to assist coding professionals and managers in decision-making processes and actions, outline expectations for making ethical decisions in the workplace, and demonstrate coding professionals' commitment to integrity during the coding process, regardless of the purpose for which the codes are being reported. The standards are relevant to all coding professionals and those who manage the coding function, regardless of the healthcare setting in which they work or whether they are AHIMA members or nonmembers.

Standards of Ethical Coding

Coding professionals should do the following:

1. Apply accurate, complete, and consistent coding practices for the production of high-quality healthcare data.

2. Report all healthcare data elements (for example, diagnosis and procedure codes, present on admission indicator, and discharge status) required for external reporting purposes (for example, reimbursement and other administrative uses, population health, quality and

patient safety measurement, and research) completely and accurately, in accordance with regulatory and documentation standards and requirements and applicable official coding conventions, rules, and guidelines.

3. Assign and report only the codes and data that are clearly and consistently supported by health record documentation in accordance with applicable code set and abstraction conventions, rules, and guidelines.

4. Query provider (physician or other qualified healthcare practitioner) for clarification and additional documentation prior to code assignment when there is conflicting, incomplete, or ambiguous information in the health record regarding a significant reportable condition or procedure or other reportable data element dependent on health record documentation (for example, present on admission indicator).

5. Refuse to change reported codes or the narratives of codes so that meanings are misrepresented.

6. Refuse to participate in or support coding or documentation practices intended to inappropriately increase payment, qualify for insurance policy coverage, or skew data by means that do not comply with federal and state statutes, regulations, and official rules and guidelines.

7. Facilitate interdisciplinary collaboration in situations supporting proper coding practices.

8. Advance coding knowledge and practice through continuing education.

9. Refuse to participate in or conceal unethical coding or abstraction practices or procedures.

10. Protect the confidentiality of the health record at all times and refuse to access protected health information not required for coding-related activities (examples of coding-related activities include completion of code assignment, other health record data abstraction, coding audits, and educational purposes).

11. Demonstrate behavior that reflects integrity, shows a commitment to ethical and legal coding practices, and fosters trust in professional activities.

Revised and approved by the House of Delegates 09/08.

Source

AHIMA House of Delegates. 2008. AHIMA Standards of Ethical Coding.

Guidelines for Achieving a Compliant Query Practice

In court, an attorney cannot "lead" a witness into a statement. In hospitals, coders and clinical documentation specialists cannot lead healthcare providers with queries. Therefore, appropriate etiquette must be followed when querying providers for additional health record information.

A query is a communication tool used to clarify documentation in the health record for accurate code assignment. The desired outcome from a query is an update of a health record to better reflect a practitioner's intent and clinical thought processes, documented in a manner that supports accurate code assignment. The final coded diagnoses and procedures derived from the health record documentation should accurately reflect the patient's episode of care.

The guidance of this practice brief augments and, where applicable, supersedes prior AHIMA guidance on queries. The intent of this practice brief is not to limit clinical communication for purposes of patient care. Rather, it is to maintain the integrity of the coded healthcare data. All professionals are encouraged to adhere to these compliant querying guidelines regardless of credential, role, title, or use of any technological tools involved in the query process.

A proper query process ensures that appropriate documentation appears in the health record. Personnel performing the query function should focus on a compliant query process and content reflective of appropriate clinical indicators to support the query.

When and How to Query

The generation of a query should be considered when the health record documentation demonstrates any of the following characteristics:

- Is conflicting, imprecise, incomplete, illegible, ambiguous, or inconsistent
- Describes or is associated with clinical indicators without a definitive relationship to an underlying diagnosis
- Includes clinical indicators, diagnostic evaluation, or treatment not related to a specific condition or procedure
- Provides a diagnosis without underlying clinical validation
- Is unclear for present on admission (POA) indicator assignment

Although open-ended queries are preferred, multiple choice and "yes/no" queries are also acceptable under certain circumstances.

To support why a query was initiated, all queries must be accompanied by the relevant clinical indicator(s) that show why a more complete or accurate diagnosis or procedure is requested. Although AHA's *Coding Clinic* for ICD-9-CM often references clinical indicators associated with

Query Example: Clarification for Specificity of a Diagnosis

Documentation:

Obtunded patient admitted with three-day history of nausea and vomiting. CXR revealed right lower lobe (RLL) pneumonia. Clindamycin ordered.

Leading query:

Is the patient's pneumonia due to aspiration?

Non-leading query:

Can the etiology of the patient's pneumonia be further specified? It is noted in the admitting history and physical examination (H&P) this obtunded patient had a history of nausea and vomiting prior to admission to the hospital and is treated with clindamycin for RLL pneumonia. Based on the above, can the etiology of the pneumonia be further specified? If so, please document the type or etiology of the pneumonia in the progress notes.

Source: AHIMA. 2011. Guidance for Clinical Documentation Improvement Programs. *Journal of AHIMA*. 81(5).

---

particular diagnoses, it is not an authoritative source for establishing the clinical indicators of a given diagnosis. A recent *Coding Clinic* issue also stated that it is not intended for such a purpose. Clinical indicators should be derived from the specific medical record under review and the unique episode of care. Clinical indicators supporting the query may include elements from the entire medical record, such as diagnostic findings and provider impressions.

A query should include the clinical indicators, as discussed above, and should not indicate the impact on reimbursement. A leading query is one that is not supported by the clinical elements in the health record or directs a provider to a specific diagnosis or procedure. The justification (that is, inclusion of relevant clinical indicators) for the query is more important than the query format.

Because the patient record should provide a sequence of events, best practice is to capture the content of a verbal or written query as well as any practitioner response to the query. This practice allows reviewers to account for the presence of documentation that might otherwise appear out of context.

If the practitioner documents his or her query response directly into the health record, and there is a lack of supporting clinical information, it is recommended the practitioner provide the clinical rationale for the diagnosis (for example, "Patient transfused four days ago due to acute blood loss anemia") unless the query is maintained as a permanent part of the health record. Lack of clinical rationale may raise questions in the event of any secondary review. Organizations that opt to not maintain queries as part of the permanent health record are encouraged to maintain copies as part of the administrative, business record. If the practitioner documents his or her response only on the query form, then the query form should become part of the permanent health record.

Choice query formats should include clinically significant and reasonable options as supported by clinical indicators in the health record, recognizing that there may be only one reasonable option. As such, providing a new diagnosis as an option in a multiple choice list—as supported and substantiated by referenced clinical indicators from the health record—is not introducing new information. Multiple-choice query formats should also include additional options, such as "clinically undetermined" and "other," that would allow the provider to add free text. Additional options, such as "not clinically significant" and "integral to," may be included on the query form if appropriate.

The "yes/no" query format should be constructed to include the additional options associated with multiple choice queries (that is, "other," "clinically undetermined," and "not clinically significant and integral to"). Yes/no queries may not be used in circumstances where only clinical indicators of a condition are present, and the condition or diagnosis has yet to be documented in the health record. Also, new diagnoses cannot be derived from a yes/no query.

In such circumstances, open-ended or multiple-choice query formats must be used. It is not considered leading to include a new diagnosis as part of a multiple choice format when supported by clinical indicators (see "Query Example: Yes/No Format"). In addition to POA determinations, yes/no queries may be utilized under the following circumstances:

- Substantiating or further specifying a diagnosis that is already present in the health record (that is, findings in pathology, radiology, and other diagnostic reports) with interpretation by a physician
- Establishing a cause and effect relationship between documented conditions, such as manifestation or etiology, complications, and conditions or diagnostic findings (for example, hypertension and congestive heart failure, diabetes mellitus, and chronic kidney disease)
- Resolving conflicting documentation from multiple practitioners

Unlike other qualifiers listed under the official coding guidelines for inpatient reporting of uncertain diagnoses, "possible" is a very broad term and therefore its use in a query is discouraged.

Query Example: Yes/No Format

Compliant Example 1

Clinical scenario: In the impression of the pathology report, ovarian cancer is documented; however, only ovarian mass is documented in the final discharge statement by the provider.

Query: Do you agree with the pathology report specifying the "ovarian mass" as an "ovarian cancer"? Please document your response in the health record or below.

Yes_____

No _____

Other _____

Clinically Undetermined _____

Name: _____ Date:_____

Rationale: This yes/no query involves confirming a diagnosis that is already present as an interpretation of a pathology specimen in the health record.

Compliant Example 2

Clinical scenario: Consulting pulmonologist documents pneumonia as an impression based on the chest x-ray. However, the attending physician documents bronchitis throughout the record, including in the discharge summary.

Query: Do you agree with the pulmonologist's impression that the patient has pneumonia? Please document your response in the health record or below.

Yes _____

No _____

Other _____

Clinically Undetermined_____

Name: _____ Date:_____

Rationale: This is an example of a yes/no query resolving conflicting practitioner documentation.

Verbal Queries and Missing Clinical Indicators

Verbal queries should contain the same clinical indicators and follow the same format as written queries to ensure compliance and consistency in policy and process. Documentation of the verbal query may be condensed to reflect the stated information but should identify the clinical indicators that support the query as well as the actual question posed to the practitioner. Verbal queries should be documented at the time of the discussion or immediately following.

The focus of external audits has expanded in recent years to include clinical validation review. The Centers for Medicare and Medicaid Services (CMS) has instructed coders to "refer to the *Coding Clinic* guidelines and query the physician when clinical validation is required."[1] The practitioner does not have to use the criteria specifically outlined by *Coding Clinic*, but reasonable support within the health record for the diagnosis must be present.

When a practitioner documents a diagnosis that does not appear to be supported by the clinical indicators in the health record, it is currently advised that a query be generated to address the conflict or that the conflict be addressed through the facility's escalation policy.

CMS recommends that each facility develop an escalation policy for unanswered queries and to address any staff concerns regarding queries. In the event that a query does not receive a professional response, the case should be referred for further review in accordance with the facility's escalation policy. The escalation process may include, but is not limited to, referral to a physician advisor, the chief medical officer, or other administrative personnel.

Query Example: Documented Conditions without Clinical Indicators

These examples provide sample wording for documentation cases that include a diagnosis without an accompanying clinical indicator.

Clinical Scenario 1

Documentation: Laboratory finding of serum sodium of 120 mmol/L and the attending physician documents hypernatremia in the final diagnostic statement.

Query: Please review the laboratory section of the present record to confirm your discharge diagnosis of hypernatremia. Laboratory findings indicate a serum sodium of 120 mmol/L.

Clinical Scenario 2

Documentation: Four-year-old child sustains a cautery injury to upper lip during maxillofacial surgery. Silvadene and dressing is applied to the affected area at the completion of the procedure, and plastic surgery was consulted. The surgeon documented in the operative report that there were "no intraoperative complications."

Query: Please review the operative note notation of "a cautery lesion to the upper lip," subsequent treatment with Silvadene, and clarify your documentation of "no intraoperative complications."

Develop Query Retention Policies

Each organization should develop internal policies regarding query retention. Ideally, a practitioner's response to a query is documented in the health record, which may include the progress notes or the discharge summary. If the record has been completed, this may be an addendum and should be authenticated. As noted in AHIMA's tool kit, "Amendments in the Electronic Health Record," "the addendum should be timely, bear the current date, time, and reason for the additional information being added to the health record, and be electronically signed."

Organizational policies should specifically address query retention consistent with statutory or regulatory guidelines. The policy should indicate if the query is part of the patient's permanent health record or stored as a separate business record. If the query form is not part of the health record, the policy should specify where it will be filed and the length of time it will be retained. It may be necessary to retain the query indefinitely if it contains information not documented in the health record. Auditors may request copies of any queries in order to validate query wording, even if they are not considered part of the legal health record.

An important consideration in query retention is the ability to collect data for trend analysis, which provides the opportunity for process improvement and identification of educational needs.

Always Follow Best Practices

Healthcare professionals that work alongside practitioners to ensure accuracy in health record documentation should follow established facility policies and procedures that are congruent with recognized professional guidelines. This practice brief represents the joint efforts of AHIMA and the Association for Clinical Documentation Improvement Specialists to provide ongoing guidance related to querying. It specifies updates to previous AHIMA practice briefs and provides support for an appropriate query process. As healthcare delivery continues to evolve, it is expected that future revisions will be required.

More Examples Online

View examples of different forms of queries (open ended, multiple choice, and so on) on the *Journal of AHIMA* website at http://journal.ahima.org and in the Query Examples given below.

Notes

1. Centers for Medicare and Medicaid Services. 2011. *Medicare Quarterly Provider Compliance Newsletter*. 1(4).

References

American Health Association. 2012. *Coding Clinic*. Second Quarter: 21.

Brown, L., P. Komara, D. Warner, L.A. Wiedemann, L. Young, eds. 2012. *Amendments in the Electronic Health Record*. Chicago: AHIMA.

AHIMA. 2010. Guidance for Clinical Documentation Improvement Programs. *Journal of AHIMA*. 81(5): 45–50.

AHIMA. 2008. Managing an Effective Query Process. *Journal of AHIMA*. 79(10): 83–88.

Query Examples

Example Verbal Query Documentation

The documentation of verbal queries should follow a standard format to include all necessary information.
Spoke with Dr. X regarding the documentation of (condition/procedure) based upon the clinical indicator(s) found in the health record (list what was found and where).

Example Open-Ended Query

A patient is admitted with pneumonia. The admitting H&P examination reveals WBC of 14,000, a respiratory rate of 24, a temperature of 102 degrees, heart rate of 120, hypotension, and altered mental status. The patient is administered an IV antibiotic and IV fluid resuscitation.

Leading: The patient has elevated WBCs, tachycardia, and is given an IV antibiotic for *Pseudomonas* cultured from the blood. Are you treating for sepsis?

Nonleading: Based on your clinical judgment, can you provide a diagnosis that represents the below-listed clinical indicators?

In this patient admitted with pneumonia, the admitting history and physical examination reveals the following:

- WBC 14,000
- Respiratory rate 24
- Temperature 102° F
- Heart rate 120
- Hypotension
- Altered mental status
- IV antibiotic administration
- IV fluid resuscitation

Please document the condition and the causative organism (if known) in the medical record.

AHIMA. 2010. Guidance for Clinical Documentation Improvement Programs. *Journal of AHIMA.* 81(5): expanded web version.

Example Multiple-Choice Query

A patient is admitted for a right hip fracture. The H&P notes that the patient has a history of chronic congestive heart failure. A recent echocardiogram showed left ventricular ejection fraction (EF) of 25 percent. The patient's home medications include metoprolol XL, lisinopril, and Lasix.

Leading: Please document if you agree the patient has chronic diastolic heart failure.

Nonleading: It is noted in the impression of the H&P that the patient has chronic congestive heart failure, and a recent echocardiogram noted under the cardiac review of systems reveals an EF of 25 percent. Can the chronic heart failure be further specified as one of the following?

- Chronic systolic heart failure_____
- Chronic diastolic heart failure_____
- Chronic systolic and diastolic heart failure_____
- Some other type of heart failure _____
- Undetermined_____

AHIMA. 2010. Guidance for Clinical Documentation Improvement Programs. *Journal of AHIMA.* 81(5): expanded web version.

Example Yes/No Queries

Compliant Example 1

Clinical Scenario: A patient is admitted with cellulitis around a recent operative wound site, and only cellulitis is documented, without any relationship to the recent surgical procedure.

Query: Is the cellulitis due to or the result of the surgical procedure? Please document your response in the health record or below.

Yes _____

No _____

Other _____

Clinically Undetermined _____

Name: _____ Date:_____

Rationale: This is an example of a yes/no query involving a documented condition potentially resulting from a procedure.

Compliant Example 2

Clinical scenario: Congestive heart failure is documented in the final discharge statement in a patient who is noted to have an echocardiographic interpretation of systolic dysfunction and is maintained on lisinopril, Lasix, and Lanoxin.

Query: Based on the echocardiographic interpretation of systolic dysfunction in this patient maintained on lisinopril, Lasix, and Lanoxin, can your documentation of "congestive heart failure" be further specified as systolic congestive heart failure? Please document your response in the health record or below.

Yes _____

No _____

Other _____

Clinically Undetermined _____

Name: _____ Date:_____

Rationale: This yes/no query provides an example of determining the specificity of a condition that is documented as an interpretation of an echocardiogram.

Compliant Example 3

Clinical scenario: During the removal of an abdominal mass, the surgeon documents, in the description of the operative procedure, a "serosal injury to the stomach was repaired with interrupted sutures."

Query: In the description of the operative procedure, a serosal injury to the stomach was noted and repaired with interrupted sutures. Can this serosal injury and repair be described by any of the following?

A complication of the procedure _____

Integral to the above procedure _____

Not clinically significant _____

Other _____

Clinically Undetermined _____

Please document your response in the health record or below accompanied by clinical substantiation.

Name: _____ Date:_____

Rationale: This is an example of a query necessary to determine the clinical significance of a condition resulting from a procedure.

Noncompliant Example 1

Clinical scenario: On admission bilateral lower extremity edema is noted; however, there are no other clinical indicators to support malnutrition.

Query: Do you agree that the patient's bilateral lower extremity edema is diagnostic of malnutrition? Please document your response in the health record or below.

Yes_____

No _____

Other _____

Clinically Undetermined _____

Name: _____ Date:_____

Rationale: Malnutrition is not a further specification of the isolated finding of a bilateral lower extremity edema. An open-ended or multiple-choice query should be used under this circumstance to ascertain the underlying cause of the patient's edema.

Noncompliant Example 2

Clinical scenario: A patient is admitted with an acute gastrointestinal bleed; the hemoglobin drops from 12 g/dL to 7.5 g/dL, and two units of packed red blood cells are transfused. The physician documents anemia in the final discharge statement.

Query: In this patient admitted with a gastrointestinal bleed and who underwent a blood transfusion after a drop in the hemoglobin from 12 g/DL on admission to 7.5 g /dL, can your documentation of anemia be further specified as an acute blood loss anemia? Please document your response in the health record or below accompanied by clinical substantiation.

Yes _____

No _____

Other _____

Clinically Undetermined _____

Name: _____ Date:_____

Rationale: In this example, a yes/no query is not appropriate for specifying the type of anemia. A multiple-choice or open-ended query is a better option.

Rationale: This query is inappropriate, as it explains the impact of the addition or removal of the diagnosis for the physician and hospital profiles. This query questions the physician's clinical judgment, which may be more appropriate in an escalation policy or physician education regarding the CDC definition of CAUTI.

Prepared by

Sandra Bundenthal, RHIA, CCS
Sue Belley, RHIA
Angie Comfort, RHIT, CDIP, CCS, CCS-P
Kathy DeVault, RHIA, CCS, CCS-P
Melanie Endicott, MBA/HCM, RHIA, CDIP, CCS, CCS-P
Cheryl Ericson, MSN, RN, CDIP, CCDS

William Haik, MD, FCCP, CDIP
Nicholas Holmes, MD, MBA
Wendy Iravedra, RHIA, CHP
Fran Jurcak, RN, MSN, CCDS
Mary Meysenburg, MPH, RHIA, CCS
Brian Murphy, CPC
Cathy Seluke, RN, BSN, ACM, CCDS
Susan Wallace, MEd, RHIA, CCS, CDIP, CCDS
Paul Weygandt, MD, JD, MPH, MBA, CCS

Acknowledgments

Bonnie Aspiazu, JD, MBA, RHIA
Dee Banet, RN, CDIP, CCDS
Jan Barsophy, RHIT
Sheila Bowlds, RHIA
Kris Brukl, RHIT
Gloryanne Bryant, RHIA, CDIP, CCS
Jane DeSpiegelaere, MBA, RHIA, CCS, FAHIMA
Rose Dunn, MBA, RHIA, CHPS, CPA, FACHE, FAHIMA
Robert Gold, MD
Garry Huff, MD
Sandra Huyck, RHIT, CCS-P
Jolene Jarrell, RHIA, CCS
Gretchen Jopp, RHIA
James Kennedy, MD, CDIP, CCS
Trey La Charite, MD
Tedi Lowjeski, RHIA, CCS, CHDA
Katherine Lusk, MHSM, RHIA
Patricia Maccariella-Hafey, RHIA, CCS, CCS-P, CIRCC
Lorie Mills, RHIT, CCS
Jennifer McCollum, RHIA, CCS
Andrea Myszewski, RHIA
Janice Noller, RHIA, CCS
Ranae Race, RHIT
Theresa Rihanek, RHIA, CCS
Laura Rizzo, MHA, RHIA
Andrew Rothschild, MD, MS, MPS, CCDS
Carol Smith
Bernice von Saleski, MAS, RHIA
Mary Webber, RHIT, CCS
Donna Wilson, RHIA, CCS, CCDS
Marna Witmer, RHIA
Gail Woytek, RHIA

Source:

AHIMA. 2013. Guidelines for Achieving a Compliant Query Practice. *Journal of AHIMA*. 84(2): 50–53.

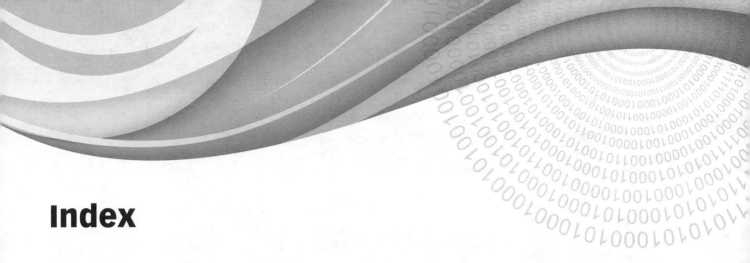

Index

Abbreviations, used in ICD-10-CM, NEC and NOS, 11

Abdominal pain, unspecified, 175

ABG results. *See* Arterial blood gas (ABG) results

ABN. *See* Advance Beneficiary Notice of Noncoverage (ABN)

Abnormal findings, 173

Abnormal weight loss/underweight, 174

Abortion

    classification of, 138

    fourth digits for, 139

    missed, 139

    resulting in live fetus, 140

Abuse

    alcohol, 56

    fraud and. *See* Fraud and abuse

    in pregnant patient, 151

Acid-fast stains, 17

Acidosis, 93

Acquired hemolytic anemias, 40–41

Acquired immunodeficiency syndrome (AIDS), 24–25. *See also* Human immunodeficiency virus (HIV)

Activity code guidelines, 194

Acute blood loss, 41

Acute bronchitis, 88

Acute hematogenous osteomyelitis, 120

Acute kidney disease, 126

Acute metabolic complications with DM, 47

Acute myocardial infarction (AMI). *See* Myocardial infarction

Acute otitis externa, 69

Acute posthemorrhagic anemia, 40, 41

Acute rheumatic fever, 74

Acute secretory OM, 70

Acute suppurative OM, 70

Acute traumatic musculoskeletal conditions, 116

Additional code

    for acute organ dysfunction, 161

    AIDS and HIV infections, 24–25

    for atherosclerosis of peripheral extremities, 82

    for chronic kidney disease, 126

    for complication of transplanted organ, 211–12

    for disorders relating to short gestation and low birth weight, 159–60

    for esophagitis, 98

    for heart failure, 75

    for hypertension, 75

    for infection of colostomy or enterostomy, 102

    infections involving bone, 131

    for kidney transplant status, 126

    for long-term use of insulin, 147

    for organism causing cellulitis, 108

    for organism causing cystitis, 127–28

    organs, 133

    for outcome of delivery, 142

    ulceration, 111

    urinary incontinence, 130

Additional diagnosis. *See also* Principal diagnosis

    for pressure ulcer stages, 110–11

    reason for surgery as, for preoperative evaluation, 4

COPD. *See* Chronic obstructive pulmonary disease (COPD)

Counseling, HIV, 25

Coxsackie virus B5, 18

CPT. *See* Current Procedural Terminology (CPT)

Crohn's disease, 101

Cross-references in Alphabetic Index, 9

Crushing injuries, 188

Cultures, specimen, 17

Cumulative effects, 197

Current burns, 189, 190

Current Procedural Terminology (CPT), changes in pattern of usage of, 232

CVA. *See* Cerebrovascular accident (CVA)

Cyanotic heart defects, 165

Cystitis, 127–28

Cystostomy, complications of, 130

DCIS. *See* Defense Criminal Investigative Service (DCIS)

Decision-making processes, 247

Decubitus (pressure) ulcer, 110–11

Deep vein thrombosis (DVT), 83

Defense Criminal Investigative Service (DCIS), 231

Deficiency anemias, 40

Degenerative joint disease (DJD), 118

Dehydration, 35

Delivery

complications of, 148–50

normal. *See* Normal delivery

outcome of, 223

preterm and postterm labor, 147

Dementia, 54

Dental codes, 98

Department of Health and Human Services (HHS), 238

HIPAA as strengthening jurisdiction of, 230

ICD-10-CM published by, 2

Derangement, chronic, old, or recurrent, 187

Dermatitis, 108–9

Diabetes mellitus (DM), 45

categories of, 46

complicating pregnancy, 49

complications and manifestations, 47

with neurological manifestations, 48

in newborns of diabetic mother, 49

with ophthalmic manifestations, 48

with other specified manifestation, 48

with peripheral circulatory disorders, 48–49

with renal manifestations, 47–48

secondary diabetes, 47

type 1, 46–47

type 2, 47

Diabetic cataract, 48

Diabetic foot ulcers, 48

Diagnoses

clarification for specificity of, 250

coding guidelines for sequencing, 4

other than disease or injury, Z codes in ICD-10-CM for reporting, 217–18

Diagnostic services, sequencing, 4

Diarrhea, definition of, 175

Digestive system, diseases of. *See* Diseases of the Digestive System (ICD-10-CM code book Chapter 11)

Direct extension, solid malignant neoplasms, 32

Disciplinary standards, enforced for compliance plan, 233

Diseases of arteries, arterioles, and capillaries, 82

Diseases of the Blood and Blood-Forming Organs (ICD-10-CM code book Chapter 3), 39–43

categories and section titles, 39

Diseases of the Circulatory System (ICD-10-CM code book Chapter 9), 73–83

categories and section titles, 73–74

Diseases of the Digestive System (ICD-10-CM code book Chapter 11), 97–104

categories and section titles for, 97

Diseases of the Ear and Mastoid Process (ICD-10-CM code book Chapter 8), 69–70

categories and section titles for, 69

Diseases of the Eye and Adnexa (ICD-10-CM code book Chapter 7), 65–66

categories and section titles for, 65

Diseases of the Genitourinary System (ICD-10-CM code book Chapter 14), 125–33

categories and section titles for, 125

Diseases of the Musculoskeletal System and Connective Tissue (ICD-10-CM code book Chapter 13), 115–21

categories and section titles for, 115–16

Diseases of the Nervous System (ICD-10-CM code book Chapter 6), 59–63

categories and section titles for, 59

Diseases of the oral cavity, salivary glands, and jaws, 98

Diseases of the Respiratory System (ICD-10-CM code book Chapter 10), 85–95

categories and section titles for, 85–86

Diseases of the Skin and Subcutaneous Tissue (ICD-10-CM code book Chapter 12), 107–12
   categories and section titles for, 107
Diseases of the tonsils and adenoids, 86
Diseases of the veins and lymphatics and other diseases of circulatory system, 83
Dislocations, 185
Disorders of appendages, 109–10
Disorders of prostate, 131
Disorders related to short gestation and low birth weight, in ICD-10-CM, 159–60
Dissociative disorders, 55
Disturbance of skin sensation, 174
Diverticular disease, 99
Diverticulosis, 99
Dizziness and giddiness, definition of, 174
DM. *See* Diabetes mellitus (DM)
Do not resuscitate (DNR) status, 224
Documentation, inadequacy of physician, 236
Documented pressure ulcer stage, 111
Dorsopathies, 119–20
Drug addiction, 56–57
Drug dependence, 56–57
Drug toxicity/hypersensitivity, 42
Drug-induced insulin coma, 49
Drug-resistant infections, 21
Drugs, adverse effects of or reactions to, 197
Duodenitis, 102
Durable medical equipment, certification of need for, 231
DVT. *See* Deep vein thrombosis (DVT)
Dysphagia, definition of, 175
Dysplasia of female organs, 133

E codes (external causes of injury and other adverse effects)
   activity, 195
   for adverse effects not classified elsewhere, 192
   for adverse effects of drugs, 197
   for burns, 189–91
   coding guidelines for, 195
   index to external causes listing, 195
   for place of occurrence, 193–94
Ear and mastoid process, diseases of, 69–70
Early satiety, definition of, 174
Eclampsia, 145
Ectopic pregnancy, 138
Eczema, 108

Education Working Party, ICD-10-AM, 235
Educational programs, developing training and, 232
EGIDs. *See* Eosinophilic gastrointestinal disorders (EGIDs)
EKGs. *See* Electrocardiograms (EKGs)
Elderly primigravida, 143
Electrocardiograms (EKGs), 77
Elevated blood pressure reading, 76
Embolism
   definition of, 82–83
   saddle, 82
Emphysema, 89
Encephalopathy, 63
Encounter for HIV screening, 25
End stage renal disease (ESRD), 126
Endocrine, Nutritional, and Metabolic Diseases (ICD-10-CM code book Chapter 4), 45–50
   categories and section titles for, 45
Endocrine system, 45
Endometriosis, classification of, 132
Enlarged prostate, 131
Enlargement of lymph nodes, 174
Enteritis, regional (granulomatous), 101
Enterobacteriaceae bacteria, 18
Eosinophilic gastrointestinal disorders (EGIDs), 100
Epilepsy, 60
Epistaxis, definition of, 174
Esophageal foreign bodies, 191
Esophagitis, fifth digits for, 98
Esophagostomy, 98
ESRD. *See* End stage renal disease (ESRD)
Estrogen receptor status, 220
Evaluations, sequencing preoperative, 4
Examinations, persons encountering health services for, 219
Excessive vomiting of pregnancy, 146
Excludes notes, 9–10
External cause status guidelines, 194
External causes of morbidity, 193
Eye and adnexa, diseases of, 65–66

Face-to-face workshops/seminars, 236
Facial weakness, 174
Factors Influencing Health Status and Contact with Health Services (ICD-10-CM code book Chapter 21), 217–26
   categories and section titles for, 217–18
Fasting plasma glucose (FPG) test, 46

Health information administration
    programs, 236
Health information management professional,
    Standards of Ethical Coding for, AHIMA,
    247–48
Health information technology program, 236
Health Insurance Portability and Accountability
    Act (HIPAA), as strengthening jurisdiction of
    DHHS, 230
Health record
    clinical indicators in, 252
    documentation, 5, 249
    use in coding process of, 11–12
Healthcare Common Procedure Coding System
    Level II codes, 237
Healthcare professionals, training in, 237
Hearing loss, sensorineural, 70
Heart defects, congenital, 164
Heart disease
    hypertension with, 75
    hypertensive, 74–75
    ischemic, 76–78
    rheumatic, 74
    valvular, 74–75
Heart failure, 78–79, 92
    diagnostic tests for, 79
    signs of, 78
Heartburn, definition of, 175
Heat, effects of, 192
Hematology, 39
Hematopoietic systems and lymphatic systems, coding
    malignancies of, 34–36
Hematuria, 129
Hemiparesis, 61
Hemiplegia, 61
Hemolytic anemias, 40
Hemolytic disease of newborn, 162
Hemophilia A. *See* Classic hemophilia
Hemophilia B. *See* Christmas disease
Hemophilia C, 42
Hemorrhage
    of digestive tract, 99, 103–4
    disorder, 42
Hemorrhagic conditions, purpura and, 42
Hepatitis
    signs and symptoms of, 24
    viral, 24
Hereditary hemolytic anemias, 40

Hernias
    abdominal, 100
    diaphragmatic (hiatal), 100
    types of, 100
Herpes simplex, 23
Herpes zoster, 23
High-risk pregnancy, prenatal supervision for, 143
HIPAA. *See* Health Insurance Portability and
    Accountability Act (HIPAA)
Hodgkin's lymphoma, 35
Human immunodeficiency virus (HIV).
    See also Acquired immunodeficiency syndrome
    (AIDS)
    codes, sequencing of, 25
    counseling, 25
    infection, 24–25, 151
Hydatid moles, 138
Hydatidiform mole. *See* Hydatid moles
Hydrocele, 131–32
Hydrocephalus, 164
Hyperemesis gravidarum, 146
Hyperplasia of prostate, 131
Hypersensitivities, 197
Hypertension, 75–76
    benign, 75
    cerebrovascular disease with mention of, 81–82
    chapter-specific coding guidelines, 75–76
    essential or NOS, 75
    gestational, 145
    heart failure caused by, 78–79
    malignant, 75
    primary, 75
    secondary, 75
    transient, 76, 145
Hypertensive cerebrovascular disease, 76
Hypertensive chronic kidney disease, 75–76
Hypertensive heart and chronic kidney disease, in
    ICD-10-CM, 75–76
Hypertensive heart disease, 75
Hypertensive retinopathy, 76
Hypertrichosis, 110
Hyperventilation, definition of, 174
Hypoglycemia, 49

ICD-10-AM Education Working Party, 235
ICD-10-CM. *See International Classification of Diseases,
    10th Revision, Clinical Modification*
    (ICD-10-CM)

Query
    generation of, 249–51
    and missing clinical indicators, verbal, 252
    retention policies, develop, 252–53
Qui tam action, 229

RA. *See* Rheumatoid arthritis (RA)
Radiation-related disorders, of skin and subcutaneous
    tissue, 109
Radiologist's findings, 173
RBCs. *See* Red blood cells (RBCs)
Reason for encounter, coding first, 3
Reason for surgery as additional diagnosis for
    preoperative evaluation, 5
Recurrence, surgical removal followed by, 36
Recurrent musculoskeletal conditions, 116
Recurrent pregnancy loss, 140
Red blood cells (RBCs), 39
    abnormal reduction of, 40
Red cell aplasia, 41
Reimbursement, impact on budgeting and, 238
Renal (kidney) disease
    chronic, 75–76, 125–26
    end-stage, 126
    hypertensive chronic, 75–76
    polycystic, 167
Renal failure, 126–27
Residual sequelae, 172
Resistance to antimicrobial drugs, 220
Respiratory conditions of fetus/newborn, 160–61
Respiratory failure and insufficiency, guidelines for
    coding and sequencing, 91–92
Respiratory infections, upper and lower, 86
Respiratory system, Z codes related to, 95
Retained foreign body fragments, 220
Retention of urine, 175
Retroperitoneal infections, 104
Rh incompatibility, 210
Rheumatic fever, acute, 74
Rheumatic heart disease, chronic, 74
Rheumatoid arthritis (RA), 117–18
Rheumatology, definition of, 116
Rib fractures, 184
Routine prenatal visits, 143
Rubella (German measles), 23
Rule of nines for burns, 190

Salivary glands, oral cavity and, 98
Salmonella gastroenteritis, 24

Schizophrenic disorders, 54
Second degree burn, 189
Secondary diabetes, 47
Secondary neoplasms, 30
Secondary thrombocytopenia, 42
Sections, format and code structure of ICD-10-CM, 7
See also cross-reference to alternative term, in
    ICD-10-CM, 9
See cross-reference to alternative term, in
    ICD-10-CM, 9
Seizures, 60, 173
Self-learning package, 235
Senile cataracts, 48
Sensorineural hearing loss, 70
Sepsis
    coding and sequencing rules for, 22–23
    septicemia and, 22
Septic shock, coding and sequencing rules for, 22–23
Septicemia and sepsis, 22
Sequencing of codes, 151–52
Serologic studies, infectious diseases diagnosed
    by, 17–18
Seventh characters, 181
Severe sepsis, coding and sequencing rules for, 22–23
Sexually transmitted diseases (STDs), 24
Shingles. *See* Herpes zoster
Sick sinus syndrome, 80
Sickle cell trait, sickle cell disease distinguished from, 40
Sickle-cell anemia, 40–41
Signs and symptoms, coding guidelines for reporting, 4
Sinus tachycardia, 81
Sinusitis, 86
Skin
    radiation-related disorders of, 109
    ulcers of, 110
SLE. *See* Systemic lupus erythematosus (SLE)
Slow fetal growth and fetal malnutrition, in
    ICD-10-CM, 160
Smear and stain examinations, 16–17
Snowflake cataract. *See* Diabetic cataract
Solid malignant neoplasms, 32
Solid tumors, 32
Somatoform disorders, 55–56
Spina bifida, 164
Spondylosis, 120
Spontaneous abortion, 139
Sporozoea, 19
Sprains, 187